Helen C. Em mott, RN
With an afterwor

D0561731

Without Regrets

A Nurse's Advice about Aging and Dying

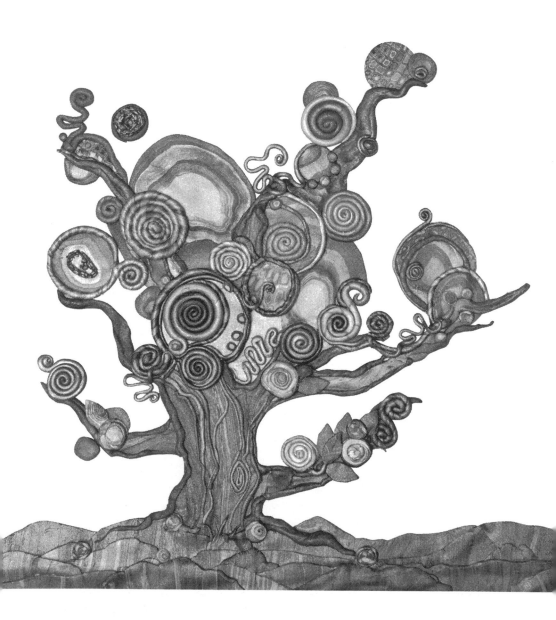

Without Regrets—A Nurse's Advice about Aging and Dying is a work of nonfiction. Persons, organizations, and events depicted in these pages are real persons and entities. All persons and stories mentioned in the text were used with permission. However, the viewpoints expressed in these stories and the lessons learned are entirely the product of the author's reflection and imagination and do not necessarily reflect the views of any organization with which the author is affiliated.

Edited by Rachel Reeder

Book design and cover tree art created by Laura Carter, Jane and Jane Design.
www.janeandjanedesign.com

Author photograph by Donna K. Blackwood

Cover art photograph by Drew Kimble, 12 Eighty-One Photography.
www.1281photo.com

Library of Congress Control Number: 2014901026

ISBN 978-0-9912759-0-8
ebook: 978-0-9912759-1-5

Published by
HCE Enterprises, LLC
121 West 48th Street, No.105
Kansas City, Missouri 66412
www.helenemmott.com

DEDICATION

*This book is dedicated to the Emmott and Clark families,
especially Isabel and Mable –
our mothers, our teachers, and our heroes.*

CONTENTS

Preface • A Nurse in the Making   vii

Introduction • First Things First
Why I Wrote This Book   15

1 • Looking back, looking forward
Goodbyes Include Grief and Celebration   27

2 • Beginning the Work
Exploring What Matters Most to Your Loved One   39

3 • Family Systems and Dynamics
A Two-edged Sword   51

4 • Choosing a Proxy Decision Maker
Who Will Be My Voice?   65

5 • Communication
Start with Being a Good Listener   81

6 • Goals of Care
The Key to Asking the Right Questions   101

7 • Caregiving
Many Roles, Many Star Players   125

8 • Choosing Mom and Dad's Last Home
Compassionate Care and Justice   145

9 • Healthcare Treatment Directives
Guidance for Proxy Decision Makers   165

Afterword • Son, Guardian, and Caregiver
A Doctor's Story, by David Emmott   187

PREFACE

A Nurse in the Making

Waiting in line to receive my diploma, thinking back over the road I had come, I asked myself, "Is this for real?" Neither of my parents had a college degree, nor did any of my nine siblings or anyone else in our family. As a kid, the eighth of ten children in a small town, I dreamed of becoming a nurse – a lofty goal – but no one doubted that I would accomplish it. It wasn't that I was smarter than the others, but I was fortunate. By the time I was growing up, many of my siblings were out and working and could lend me a hand. Early on I also had a bit of charisma, that is, a blend of grit and humor that endeared family and friends to me. When I said I wanted to become a nurse, their love and support was the strength I needed to overcome all obstacles.

I remember the first time that I actually met and got to know a nurse. Darlene wore a starched white uniform and a hat like the one Sally Field wore in the Flying Nun television show. I babysat for Darlene's three small children the summer after seventh grade. I stayed with her the entire summer, about thirty miles from my hometown. Her husband was in Vietnam. She impressed me because she was upright in stature and so very professional looking as she left for work each day.

During high school, I worked after school in a doctor's office. His wife had a bachelor's degree in nursing. The doctor and his wife thought I was very bright. I wasn't sure, but honestly? I did think I was much smarter than the doctor's wife. That seems funny now, but I was obviously watching other people and gathering information that would further my goal of becoming a nurse. I worked in that office for several years, even after graduating from high school, but I never veered far from plans to attend college.

At the age of twenty-two, I made my way to the University of Oklahoma. I took seventeen or more hours each semester, working two jobs much of the time. I loved learning and making new friends. I had a goal in sight – I was going to be a nurse.

My toughest hurdle was chemistry. I had poor preparation from my small-town high school. Then I met David Emmott, a medical student, who agreed to tutor me. I went quickly from a C average to a brush at getting an A. In the end, I settled happily for a B because I had also met the love of my life. David fell for me, he reports, because I was hard working and honest, two things he hadn't seen a lot of in the sorority girls he had been dating. I'll never forget walking across the stage and being handed my diploma. Many of my brothers and sisters, along with Mom and Dad, attended the ceremony. Their presence meant everything to me. Dad even paid for a huge luncheon for everyone afterwards. He was so conservative with his money. I knew then that he shared my joy. I was on cloud nine. A bachelor's degree in nursing was a good beginning toward a promising career in healthcare.

David and I married during his third year of medical school. We had very little money as I had to finish my nursing degree while he was finishing medical school. Still, it sounds like a fairy tale, and maybe it was. Our backgrounds were so different. We were an unlikely match. Yet, I was really good at the things he wasn't and vice versa. He taught me to play tennis, backgammon and gin rummy, only to find that eventually I would beat him handily at all three. I could finish all the biblical questions in the *New York Times* crossword puzzle, make terrific pies, and make him laugh when he was dead tired from his training to become a doctor. The honest truth is that we were both from such big families that having one another was truly what we needed. Unconditional love and strong Midwestern values fueled our journeys to build our family and finish David's training.

We moved to Kansas City from Oklahoma. David began his urology residency. I worked in an out-patient doctor's office for a short time. I was terrible at making the doctor's coffee. The move to Kansas City was thirty-two years ago. In fact, David, will be taking his Urology Boards, required every ten years, for the third and final time, very soon.

My career in nursing didn't quite turn out the way I planned. Early in my career, I worked in pediatric intensive care units, including stints in the neonatal and burn units at a children's hospital. Eventually I returned to hospital work in an intensive care unit for adults. That is where the work of a nurse began to sting. Day after day, taking care of critically ill patients was hard. The distress of working in an environment where patients were critically ill and dying while their families sat alone in dismal waiting rooms was hard for me. Doctors could be arrogant and even irrational if I questioned their orders or called them in the night.

My unrest caused me to doubt the calling that I had felt so naturally when younger. There were many nights when getting into my car to return home, I actually hoped that I or one of the kids would get sick so I wouldn't have to return the next morning. It was more than fatigue. It was frustration with how patients were aggressively treated, regardless of their prognosis. Saving lives at all costs was the norm in the intensive care unit, but it didn't seem right to me.

After we had a third child and David began a private practice, I became a full-time mother and housewife. I quickly became restless. What about studying something in the humanities? Reading and thinking about things that I had never had time to ponder might be fun. What about dabbling in some philosophy courses? I read Plato's *Republic*, took classes on the history of knowledge, learned to write essays about rationalism, learned to spell epistemology, and fell in love with ethics courses taught by a German professor at the University of Missouri in Kansas City.

My nursing background and love for knowledge was the perfect fit for studying with Dr. Uffelmann. He called me a veteran of the station wagon and adored the fact that I often scored higher on tests than the medical students. Years later, I learned that I probably had more hours in his class rooms than anyone because he was such a tough professor. He actually gave one of my classmates an *F minus*. He didn't frighten me. He was not much different from doctors with whom I had worked, or my dad, who was a minister, or for that matter, my father-in-law, a physician with a booming voice. I knew I could not only survive Dr. Uffelmann's challenging classes but learn what was important and "right" and "wrong" about our healthcare system.

Dr. Uffelmann was one of three founders of an ethics center in Kansas City. The organization was doing groundbreaking work in end-of-life care, children's rights, and patients' rights, generally. They held town hall meetings regarding allocation of healthcare funds and talked about rationing of healthcare. I became a groupie. Eventually I requested to do an internship at the ethics center under Dr. Uffelmann's guidance. Ethics felt like the Cinderella slipper that I had been in search of for many years.

For the next decade, I drove my kids to soccer games, ballet, and all the other things young families do. I traveled to Haiti to do charitable work, volunteered at a pediatric clinic for uninsured children, and earned a degree in philosophy, receiving departmental honors. I found I could use my head in philosophy and ethics and practice kindness and compassion at the clinic and on my trips to Haiti – a perfect balance for my career and personality.

I look back now and see that I was trying to carve out a niche for myself in which vulnerable people would be treated with human dignity and given a chance to know their rights and participate actively in decisions about their healthcare treatments – so unlike the top-down care I had recently witnessed in intensive care units.

My graduate paper for a master's degree in bioethics and healthcare policy was a "Personal Review and Justice Analysis of Nursing Experiences in Haiti." It was later published in the *Journal for the Poor and Underserved*. In this paper I conclude that nurses and doctors are not only morally better off working to bring about justice, but our profession demands that we do such things. If not, we become parts of a bigger problem and avoid the moral obligations that are at the core of our profession.

Along the way, while studying, volunteering, and working on ethics projects, David and I and our three children grew up together. I call us a medical family. I use that term because we are the family that our relatives rely on to help them make decisions about their health; we are also the "go to" family for friends whose kids or parents are sick. Our door has always been open to be of help and our phones ring at all hours of the night. There really is no end to the ways family and friends have needed help translating the ins and outs of healthcare over many of the last thirty years.

I currently teach part-time at a university in a theology department. I teach courses focused on applied healthcare ethics and theories addressing the many difficult decisions in healthcare. I find great peace in passing on my past experiences with the sick and vulnerable in hospitals and Haiti. I love giving students tools to help them advocate for their loved ones or teach others how to navigate illness, frailty, and dying.

Earlier in my career I believed that children in intensive care units, people in Haiti, and uninsured and sick children in my own community were the most vulnerable humans I would encounter, but I was wrong. Our mothers' final years of life exemplified a state of vulnerability I could not have imagined. David and I learned when helping them how challenging decision making and caregiving for aging parents can be – even for a doctor and a nurse.

We survived a sick child, the loss of one of our children's friends to a house fire, the deaths of both of our fathers and other bumps in the road of life. Life was full of lessons that seemed to only prepare us for the next step. Along the journey, we had much to celebrate: a thriving practice for David, recovered health for our son, amazingly smart and loving children, who loved each other and us. Add to the journey, ten years of the realities we faced caring for our mothers, and, as an already seasoned medical family, we had many new tools to add to the arsenal of life and death experiences. Those years were stacked full of life lessons that I – no we – are willing to pay forward by sharing our heartfelt stories and our friends' stories in the pages of this book.

Helen Emmott, RN, MA
October 16, 2013

ACKNOWLEDGMENTS

Words cannot express how grateful I am for all the families and friends who shared their stories with me and allowed me to include their stories in these pages. Many of their parents' completed their journeys before I finished the book. I thank the Center for Practical Bioethics for its pioneering role in advance care planning and for helping me become a nurse ethicist. Thanks also to my amazing husband David and my friend and mentor Myra Christopher, for believing in me always – more times than I can count – and to the William F. O'Connor Foundation in Chicago and the Shepherd's Center, Central in Kansas City, Missouri, for trusting me with their resources.

INTRODUCTION

First Things First
Why I Wrote This Book

The content in this book is inspired by my family and my husband's family: two very different families living very different scenarios and making very different choices at the end of life. Mable, my mother, was a farm woman; Isabel, David's mother, was a Canadian aristocrat. My mother had presence of mind until the very end of her life; David's mother had dementia for several years. My father didn't believe much in science or medicine; David's father was a surgeon.

David and I did not anticipate becoming responsible for the care of our aging parents. Who among us thinks of old age, dying, or closure in the middle of building a career and family? Who is clear-sighted enough to realize that as we are just beginning to hit our stride, our elders are slowing down, their biological clocks ticking away, and their health status changing?

But as the Emmott children grew up, so our parents aged, and we spent the next decade caring for family and making decisions. The responsibilities were often overwhelming. Though our professions – I am a nurse ethicist and David is a physician – focus on teaching others to make healthcare decisions, we had to learn first-hand the challenges involved in helping our parents and families imagine and live the final chapters of their lives. Early in the experience, I began to see that other couples and most families will, sooner or later, encounter the same challenges and need to build the same expertise, though each family must find its own way.

This book grew out of my desire to share the benefits and insights that we gained along the way. We learned many lessons, from each other, from other family members and from our friends and patients who also shared their stories with us. As we continue to reflect on our experience, talk with our friends, and work with other professionals doing end-of-life planning, we realize how important it is to engage one another in this conversation. In our decade of caring, we did some things well, some things not so well. We fell down at times, but we always got back up. We tried to hold dear and respect the lives of our loved ones. We tried to

Though our professions focus on teaching others to make healthcare decisions, we had to learn first-hand the challenges involved in helping our parents and families imagine and live the final chapters of their lives.

accept – and help them accept – the inevitable losses that accompany extreme age and frailty, and to tread on with courage.

So this book is not about perfect solutions. I hope that by reading this book you will be better prepared than David and I were to become caregivers, companions and comforters for your loved ones. I hope that your experience with frail or dying family members or friends will not be so burdensome that you become sick or that your family comes undone. But mostly, I hope that you will learn to make decisions with and for your loved ones with confidence. When you begin to look back on this process, I hope that you will be able to do so with no regrets.

There is no way to anticipate the situations families will encounter when caring for aging parents or loved ones, or how they will respond to those encounters. No formula exists for making the decisions easy or predictable. But this book can help you work through such "stuff" – the stuff all families go through when a parent or spouse becomes frail or disabled, or loses the capacity to make his or her own decisions.

Sometimes the way forward has been anticipated, discussed or even preplanned and just needs tweaking. Sometimes the whole terrain lies unmapped before us. So what did David and I do? What should you do? I will try to unfold that in the chapters to come. First, however, I would like you to meet my mother. I can feel her presence on my shoulder, reminding me to tell you something important.

A singular woman

In 1986, after fifty-four, yes fifty-four, years of marriage, my mom, Mable Clark, divorced my dad, the reverend Joe Clark. She had decided that time was running out for her. She had some things that she needed to do. A large crack appeared in the Clark family because, apparently, it was Mother's turn to call the tune. That same year, I diapered a new baby, rode herd on two toddlers, and set up house in a better part of town as my husband David built his surgical practice. As my mother reclaimed her long-lost independence, I watched mine go down the drain. I was busy figuring out what the world expected of me, unaware that my mother had already been there and done that. I was also unaware that as she reclaimed control of her life, she would also claim control of her dying and motivate me to write about it.

Sometimes the way forward has been anticipated, discussed or even preplanned and just needs tweaking. Sometimes the whole terrain lies unmapped before us.

Mable Clark was one tough cookie – as tough as nails on the outside and gentle as a lamb on the inside. She raised ten children while fulfilling all the real and imagined duties of a minister's wife. She smacked and switched every one of us at one time or another. I remember vividly the time I was subjected to the "go and choose your own switch" routine. I had been hanging the younger ones' diapers on the clothes line, wrinkled, and using only one clothes pin.

Another time when I was a young teen, I called her on the phone and yelled at her. "I hate you," I told her. "I swear you never listen to me." She drove all the way down Main Street to smack my face – almost before I could hang up the phone. Yet, only seventy-two hours later, she placed a note in the church bulletin announcing that she would be making and selling pies for the next two weeks – including coconut and banana cream pies and fruit pies using fruit she had canned over the summer. Only she and I knew the pie money would be used to buy fabric to make a dress for me to wear to a high school event. And she told no one that the event would include dancing, something that we were strictly forbidden to do. Whenever any one of us recalls a "tough" Mable story, it is just as quickly followed by a "gentle, tender" Mable story.

In Mother's younger days, she never rested. She was selfless and spent her life helping others. She cooked, cleaned, gardened, washed clothes, canned food, and sewed clothing and drapes, all while holding down jobs that required hard physical labor. I wonder now how she did all the things she did. She was active in the church community, tended her children, and lived with our Dad as his chosen profession dictated she should live.

Sunday mornings, I awakened before dawn to the clanging of pots and pans. Several hours later, when I finally got to the kitchen myself, the windows were always steamy. Pots of black-eye peas, new potatoes, fried okra, over-cooked pot roast, and other Sunday staples simmered on all the burners. On many Sundays, she had already fried chicken and made biscuits by 7 A.M.

She had only two dresses, and they were identical except for their color. One was blue; the other, pink. As a young girl, she let me choose the one she would wear to church on Sunday morning. We followed this routine numerous times but always pretended that it was a novel experience. Then, off to church we would go, all ten of us knowing that we could invite a friend home after church, and knowing that our friends would come. They didn't come because we were cool or popular or had a tidy house, but because they knew my mother's cooking and the spontaneous chaos they would enjoy at the Clark home until we were hauled back to church for the evening service.

One by one, my older siblings married and fled the constraints of Dad's fundamentalist interpretation of the Bible – "no dancing, no shorts, no make-up, no playing cards, and no movies" were some of the injunctions he made us follow. One-by-one, we younger kids were left behind. We lived for holidays and other occasions when our older brothers and sisters returned to shower presents and attention on Mom and the rest of us.

Mom loved her sons- and daughters-in-law as much or more than her own children. She discovered their favorite foods and included them in our lavish holiday dinners. I once asked her how she knew if her children had chosen the right spouses. She answered, "If my children like them, I like them. If my children love them, I love them." Divorces occurred in some of these early marriages, but Mom never divorced the departing in-law. Her love and loyalty were unfailing.

In 1986, we knew things would never be the same – that's how each of us interpreted the big divorce. Some of my siblings had experienced their own divorces; some were too busy to worry. But, worried or not, we all cried.

Mom set about discovering herself in many ways. She bought a new car and ventured to New Mexico to visit her only surviving sister. She lived in Arkansas and Oklahoma for a while, and was a home companion for elders who were only a few years older than she. She came to Kansas City and watched the Kansas City Royals play ball, and finally chose to reside in Kansas City. She made our friends her friends and even our friends' parents became her friends. Instead of cooking for us on holidays, we cooked for her. And, over time, instead of taking care of us, we began taking care of her.

Eventually, Mom decided that she needed to move to an assisted living residence. She was very proud of her "suite." She furnished it with a small sofa, lots of romance novels, and photographs of all her children and grandchildren. She loved getting manicures, being served three meals a day at a table with cloth napkins, playing bingo, and listening to volunteer singers perform old church hymns and country songs. She acted like a queen, and in fact, she was elected queen during the festivities on Valentine's Day. She wore her tiara for weeks.

Her final residence was in a nursing facility where she soon became the favorite of all the nurses and aides who cared for her. She was funny and feisty and always had a smile on her face. I, on the other hand, was sad and teary eyed. It distressed me to see her living in a nursing home. "You really should come to my home and live with me," I cried. But she would grin, look at me with her big blue eyes, and say, "I like it here. Go home." I never knew if she was being honest or only telling me what I needed to hear.

Those of us who were part of Mom's last twenty years received a glorious gift. We watched her spread her wings and find herself while she was still able to do so. We revisited the past with all its ups and downs and were able to say "I'm sorry." She said, "I'm sorry, too." And, in the final years when we told her we loved her, she always said "I love you, too." We seldom heard these words when we were kids.

In Mom's dying days, our family became the way it was when we were young. We rallied together and said our "goodbyes" in whatever ways we could manage. Some said their goodbyes over the phone, others were at the bedside. We sang songs with the hospice chaplain and let her grandchildren and great-grandchildren crawl on her bed. We laughed. We cried. It was hard work. It wasn't pretty. It felt like we were delivering her into a new life as she had delivered each of us into life in this world.

On her last day, I asked to have some time alone with her. I told her that I loved her. I thanked her for teaching me how to be a good mother and to have a positive outlook on life. I told her that I didn't really know what heaven would be like, but I knew that others were waiting there for her. I laughed and cried at the same time when I told her that Dad would be perfect in heaven, and she might even fall in love with him again!

As I prepared my mother's eulogy, it was undeniable that Mable Clark had sacrificed much over the years as a minister's wife and the mother of ten children. And, still somehow, she had lived and died on her own terms.

As a high school student and young adult, I had thought myself smarter and more chic than my mother. I took Geometry and Algebra. She had only an eighth-grade education. She made her own mayonnaise. I bought mine at a gourmet grocery store. She didn't even have her own check book!

In my childhood, Dad had stood at the front of the grocery store and smoked a cigar while mother filled the grocery cart. When all the coupons were redeemed and all the groceries bagged, he strolled to the register and wrote the check. He wouldn't let her visit her two sisters because they had married and divorced more times than we could count. I went to college. I got an education, thinking it would liberate me from the dull roles rural America had assigned to women like my mother. Her lack of independence suffocated me.

But after her divorce, Mom opened her own checking account and visited her "wayward" sister. She sold the big Oldsmobile that Dad had given her and bought a small sports car! But more than that, she let her children know what was important to her. She told us what she valued, what her final years would look like, and how she wanted to die. I began to realize that her life exemplifies a type of wisdom that only comes from journeying open-eyed and joyful through ninety-five years of life.

Sharing Mother's story

The year Mom died, I taught a college course for senior nursing students introducing them to the topic of advance care planning. I told them that a person's life story can help us know how a person wants to die. Time and again, I found myself using my mother as an example. Her diligent preparation and willingness to communicate with us kids were strong examples of how advance directives can extend a person's independence well beyond his or her ability to remain independent.

Many of the students argued that their grandparents were old school and didn't want to talk about intimate topics such as how they want to be treated when they can no longer care for their own bodies or how they want to die. One student talked about how overwhelmed her dad was, when his mother (the student's grandmother) said she was leaving all such decisions to him. One student told the class about her brother's death from AIDS and how her parents had disregarded the values and concerns of his life partner. In response to their trepidation, I told them about my mother. I said, "Yes, your grandmother can talk about her wishes. Listen to this story about my mother. Listen to stories about my husband's family, my friends' families, and my patients' experiences. They will help you. They will teach you. They will make you feel normal. They will make you laugh. They will make you cry. But, most of all, you will benefit from them."

I told them that a person's life story can help us know how a person wants to die. Time and again, I found myself using my mother as an example.

I urged them to collect similar stories from their own families and to listen to the stories their friends told. I knew that such stories would prepare them to understand and recognize the gravity of the challenges they would face when, as healthcare providers, they were called to support dying patients and their families.

Then, as part of their assignment, I required that each student complete an advance directive. I asked them, that is, to explore their values, and document the kind of healthcare they would want to receive if they were involved in a traumatic and potentially disabling accident or after receiving a terminal diagnosis. I also asked them to explain their decisions to one or more of the other students.

My mother's story caught their imagination, and in the weeks that followed, various students began to speak openly about the encounters and conversations they had initiated with their parents, grandparents, spouses, and even roommates as a result of this assignment. They had gotten it! The gulf between life and learning narrowed. Then and only then, did I connect my mother's wisdom with the knowledge that I had long been attempting to convey to my students.

And, so, my mom is with me today, always encouraging me, and always serving as a model of newfound independence. She was in her seventies when she pursued her freedom. With few resources and little education, she reclaimed her life from her married identity. She lived without regrets those last twenty years. Who could have imagined such a transformation?

Do all American families have the resolution and clarity about life that my family attained? I sincerely doubt it. In fact, I know that they do not. I know some families who have never gotten along or agreed about anything and others who ignore or totally deny looming health issues. Still others may focus on financial resources like savings or insurance, seemingly unaware of or immune to the difficulties that lurk behind even the best financial securities. Estate planning can be very important, but this book is about relationships, living well, and dying as Mable Clark did, as freely as she had lived.

Looking ahead

Each of the chapters in this book tells a story (or stories) to help us successfully accompany and care for aging or frail parents, spouses, or friends. The lessons we learn from the stories accumulate with each chapter. Some will be more useful to you than others, but you will gain important information from each of them. Applying these lessons to your own life can help you and your family make better choices and avoid confusion. In this introduction I have told my mother's story as a way to begin the conversation. Don't be surprised, however, if Mable also finds her way into other chapters. Her no nonsense approach to life and dying delights me even now.

Chapter One addresses the tensions and inevitable transitions in our relationships that accompany the end of life, the pull on our minds and hearts when grief and celebration are entwined. The simple but profound truth that emboldens care is being able to value what remains: grief and death are not the end of our relationships.

Chapter Two describes how your parents' values and beliefs influence their declining years and their healthcare decisions as they get older and become more dependent. I will also offer some tips on how you can begin conversations that will help them explore these delicate topics.

Chapter Three explores family dynamics and the importance of understanding how your family works in both positive and negative ways. David and I have fifteen siblings between us but we know that "only children" have challenges, too.

Chapter Four emphasizes the importance of choosing a proxy, that is, a surrogate decision maker or power of attorney for healthcare decisions. What characteristics make one a good proxy? How do parents determine whom to ask, and what questions ought the proxy ask his or her parents? What should they expect their role to be?

Chapter Five addresses communication issues that an individual will confront when he or she accepts the role of caregiver or healthcare proxy.

Chapter Six includes valuable lessons about establishing goals of care for aging family members.

Chapter Seven focuses on caregiving from both the cared for and the caregiver's points of view. I will also ask you to consider what can happen if the caregiver's health and well-being are neglected or compromised.

Chapter Eight confronts the challenges you will face in choosing where your parents will reside during their declining years, the difficulties of caring for them at home, and how you can anticipate future decisions if remaining at home becomes unsafe or untenable for various reasons.

Chapter Nine explores the choices that must be made when aging parents experience serious illness. This chapter is a complement to chapter 4. In that chapter, we discussed the formal appointment of a healthcare proxy. In this chapter, we discuss the use of the healthcare treatment document as a guide to hearing your parents' voices and acting on their wishes. Together, an involved and loving family and an informed healthcare proxy can partner with the healthcare team – to insure that your parents avoid defaulting to a medical glide path that almost always makes a standard of aggressive curative care their only choice.

And so I write, and have written, to invite you to talk openly and honestly with your parents about their values, their hopes, their ideas of how they want to die. It is their journey; accompanying them and giving voice and substance to their decisions is your privilege.

The poet Mary Oliver writes in "When the Roses Speak, I Pay Attention":

. . . "Listen,
the heart-shackles are not, as you think
death, illness, pain,
unrequited hope, not loneliness, but
lassitude, rue, vainglory, fear, anxiety,
selfishness."

I write, and have written, to give you courage and resolve so that when the journey is finished, your grief will not be heavy and no regrets will shackle your heart.

CHAPTER 1

Looking Back, Looking Forward
Goodbyes Include Grief and Celebration

Yesterday I went to visit a close friend of mine who is dying. I'll call her P. That's how she always marked her golf balls – with a huge blue P. She was diagnosed with advanced bladder cancer only ten days ago and went from a diagnostic stay in a local hospital to an in-patient hospice house. She had known she was sick for a long time, but had chosen to deny it as long as possible. Now she chose to forgo any life sustaining treatments. Her best friend and husband had died unexpectedly from a heart attack in his late fifties. For twenty years, she had worn her wedding ring on a chain around her neck. I am a nurse. I have seen death, even deaths of small children in intensive care units. And I watched my mother die an inch at a time from mere aging and frailty. But this woman was my golfing buddy.

When I arrived she teased me and called me Emmott as she always had. No one else has called me that since I was a young pup in nursing school. We laughed as we remembered forty dollars she had never let me pay her, the result of a disastrous gin rummy game when we were on a golf trip several years ago. We laughed, but she was dying, and I knew instantly that this death was different.

I wasn't prepared for this tough and independent peer to be gray in color, with gurgling noises coming from her throat, and fluids leaking from her mouth and nose. I cleaned her face with a cool, soapy cloth. I cried. She moaned as I repositioned her head. I had watched my mother's health status diminish over a period of years. She lost her ability to read, hear, or communicate; essentially, she became unable to find significant meaning in her daily life. I was better prepared to say "goodbye" to Mom than to this close friend whose death was sudden.

This time it hurts. This is how acute grief looks, feels, and smells. I didn't want to leave her side but knew I should. I tried to say "goodbye" but said instead, "See you later, Powell," as I backed out the door. I felt an overwhelming sadness.

Honoring the spirit

A few years before my mother died, as I was completing my master's degree in bioethics, I interned with a hospice chaplain who specialized in geriatrics. I made rounds with "Rev Beck" at a traditional nursing home and accompanied her on home visits to many aging clients. I had known Beck for years through a faith community and the bioethics center, but this quiet and demure woman, who wore a religious collar, packed a pastoral punch like nothing I had ever seen before. When she entered patients' rooms or homes, it felt almost as though a light surrounded her entire being. She was literally transformed!

She touched each patient's hand, and straightforwardly but softly asked, "How's your spirit today?"

She touched each patient's hand, and straightforwardly but softly asked, "How's your spirit today?" Even those with advanced memory issues or patients who were actively dying from cancer and other diseases heard her ask: "How's your spirit, Bessie?" "Tell me how your spirit is today, Mr. Jones." Patiently, she listened to stories about loneliness, cancer, and general loss of health. She addressed their hardships and promised communication with families and staff. At the end of each visit, she always asked if she could sing for them, literally, a song of their choice. I heard Beatles' tunes, Irish tunes, sweet and tender hymns, and watched patients and families laugh and cry. Rev Beck could really sing! Many patients sang along with her – even those with dementia.

On one occasion, a very elderly African-American woman named Thelma asked Beck to sing a tune Beck didn't know. I was paralyzed. I not only knew the tune, I knew every word to "Pass Me Not, O Gentle Savior." It was my turn to give. I held Thelma's hand and recalled the song from my early years in the Baptist church. She sang

Call them by name. Ask them about their pain. Ask them about their past. Ask them about their spirit and what they hope for.

with me. Tears ran down my face. I learned that day a tiny bit about the art of tending to those who are at the end of their journeys. And, collectively, over the semester, I learned how important it is to acknowledge each patient as a valuable human being: Call them by name. Ask them about their pain. Ask them about their past. Ask them about their spirit and what they hope for.

Beck pointed out to me that aging itself is a type of grieving, a time of change, and change nearly always includes loss. My Grandmother Clark quit eating and drinking in her final days. With her hearing and vision horribly impaired, she saw her physical realm disappearing inch by inch, year by year. Eventually Grandma's life was almost empty of all the things that had given it meaning. Her six daughters had died before her. Cutting off her long, braided hair became her tipping point, the final loss.

Each aging person is unique. The things in life that give them happiness, meaning, joy, and hope are different for each person. My mother may have been a deeply spiritual person but she had such a "no nonsense" attitude about life that I had never really talked with her about her beliefs in things beyond this world. Mom was more of a doer than a talker. After my time with Rev Beck, I decided to try and have a conversation with Mom about deeper things. I thought I would check on her spirit as I had witnessed Rev Beck do to other similarly aging women and men.

One day as we sat in the atrium at Sharon Lane Nursing Home, I asked her, "So, Mom, how's your spirit?" I was ready for a moving conversation. I thought I would encourage her and maybe sing her a song. Mom looked sternly at me and said, "Well. That's really none of your business. How's yours?" I laughed so hard I almost fell over. Tears of joy. Tears of relief. At that moment, I was Mom's daughter, not her caregiver and not her chaplain. Even when I feared that each visit might be our last, there were opportunities to celebrate and enjoy the moment – not every visit had to be overtly serious, deep, and end in soulful singing.

Grieving and celebrating what is, while it is

On a recent Sunday when David was on call, I walked to a church near our condo in search of inspiration. To my surprise, the theme for the morning service was laughter! Instead of a sermon or a homily prepared by one of the regular ministers, a visiting comedian was in the pulpit. She was probably seventy years-old and told us that before her career in comedy and humor, she had been a school teacher. I was skeptical at first, but soon found myself not only laughing but learning about the many benefits of laughter. As she entertained us she also informed us about the many physiological changes that occur as we laugh. She said that she had spent the last decade traveling the world and presenting her program to patients and healthcare professionals, simultaneously teaching and provoking laughter. She wanted us to know that laughter has healing powers so tremendous that there is only a fine line between laughing and crying.

As I listened to her, I also recalled how many times Mom and I had bouts of giddiness even as her health declined. I remembered that even when she was actively dying my sisters and I sometimes behaved like silly teenagers, teasing one another, laughing and watching to see if Mom would acknowledge our rowdiness as she had when we were younger. As we faced her impending death, we were unknowingly healing our bodies and souls by laughing and crying – by grieving and celebrating.

As we faced her impending death, we were unknowingly healing our bodies and souls by laughing and crying – by grieving and celebrating.

I admit that I felt a sweet sense of relief when Mom took her final breath. And even now after several years, my emotional pendulum still swings from celebrating memories to grieving her absence. This woman I had not been close to until my forties had become my best friend, my teacher, my raison d'etre. There was a correlation between obtaining my degree in philosophy at age forty and finding peace with how my mother and I related to each other. I had always felt that I was smarter than Mom, but I learned in my forties that book smarts was a privilege that not everyone had. I also learned that being wise wasn't always easy and that wisdom presents itself in funny ways and often comes from people who are easily overlooked.

A different kind of presence

The day Mable Clark died, I felt empty. I wondered if the loss I felt so keenly would ever become a lighter burden. And I wasn't even clear about how I really felt. I was relieved that she was not suffering, or stuck in a life she could no longer enjoy or share with others, which was the true foundation of her being. Most of all, I missed her. The year following her death was time I would need to figure out what had happened and how my mother's living and dying had shaped my life. I quickly learned that though her physical presence was absent, I could still hold her near and dear to my heart, speak freely about what she had taught me, and honor some of what she had taught me by writing this book.

> *I wondered if the loss I felt so keenly would ever become a lighter burden.*

There is an ancient sarcophagus from the Northern Wei Dynasty on display at the Nelson-Atkins Museum in Kansas City that, like many Chinese and Egyptian tombs, teaches a series of moral lessons about filial piety. The stories are engraved on panels. The story that most impressed me was about a young boy who was devoted to his grandfather. One scene shows the young boy and his father putting the older man on a gurney that the young man had been instructed to build. The boy and his father then carry him to the top of a hill to leave him.

We asked the art docent leading our tour if they were abandoning the old man because he was sick. She told us that the family in the story had fallen on hard times and the old man had become useless and unproductive. A subsequent scene shows the father and son walking away, leaving the older man behind. The son reaches for the gurney, but his father tells him to leave it there. "But,

Father," said the son, "Won't I need this gurney to bring you here one day?" The final scene is of the three of them, returning down the hill toward home.

Many times while writing this book, I have thought about that sarcophagus, the ultimate lesson of caring for an elder, the revelation that the role of elders is not over when their physically productive years are past. The story also reveals that how we love and respect our parents greatly influences the way our children will care for us in our time of aging.

I have always loved Joan Didion's writings. Most recently, she has written books about her husband's and her daughter's deaths, which occurred very close to one another. Her husband John Dunne died suddenly one evening of a massive heart attack shortly after they returned from visiting their daughter Quintana in the hospital. Quintana subsequently recovered and married, but then she, too, died suddenly, leaving Joan doubly bereaved. Joan described John's death and her grief in *The Year of Magical Thinking*. She described her experience and emotions so powerfully that I lost track of whose loss I was grieving. I imagined my own husband dying or the death of one of my children. But, as Didion writes, such grief is finally unreal and unimaginable. One cannot truly know how it feels until it smacks you in the face.

Our immediate experience of grief, she points out, is somewhat muted by the press of events: the autopsy if there is one, the funeral, the rituals of saying goodbye. She points out that those incidents paper over the hardest part of grief. The real challenge is how we face the voids, the absence of that person in all the life events that we were accustomed to sharing with them. In Didion's world, grief can never make sense. It is absurd, a void, a missing person, the opposite of presence, purpose, meaning.

It has been over three years since Mom died. I have a picture of her setting on my dressing table. My son Cameron and I are also in this picture, which was taken the summer before she died. I see her sitting there each day. She looks tiny in the picture but I remember her as larger than life. She was large in the spirit she didn't want to talk about and even bigger in knowing how to live a good and meaningful life. Even when Mom was alive, I always wished for her presence whenever I found something beautiful, like the mountains in Colorado or lavender fields in southern France. Her life had been tough. She hadn't had many opportunities to travel, relax, or enjoy the good things of life. Now these thoughts and feelings are magnified. When I enjoy a great meal that reminds me of her, I fight back tears. When I use her old, tattered cookbook and see her handwriting in the margins describing how to make the recipes even better, I laugh and cry. What a great woman my Mom was!

Joan Didion wrote that in the year after she lost her husband, she saved his shoes. He would come back and need them, her imagination informed her, though she knew that such thinking was more magical than real. We must eventually, as she writes later in the book, resolve to let the dead be dead. We keep them alive so we won't have to walk alone. But at some point I must let go. I know how hard it can be.

A final belief that comes to us from ancient times, whether from biblical Israel, Greek, Egyptian, Chinese, or other cultural tradition, is that we can honor those who have gone before us even after their lives on earth have ended. I hope that this book trumps all things said and unsaid to my mother, so that I can finally celebrate her life more than grieve her absence.

Mom never stopped teaching me the uniqueness of human beings and their spirits. I think the most important thing I learned from watching Mom die is that her death was hers, not mine – just as her life had been hers and not mine. I can still shed tears but I can't sit in the puddle. I still have things to do, and many of these are things she taught me to do: love my children and grandchildren, teach them about success and sorrow, and pick them up when they stumble.

I experienced a newfound peace when I gave my mother's eulogy at her funeral. I am the eighth of ten children, one of the babies and one of the short ones. But with humility and hope, I addressed an audience of over one hundred at a Baptist church, the very religion Mom and I had both fled. I believe that people were shocked that I had been chosen to speak. I found strength in thinking about Mom and how much she, too, had surprised some of these same individuals in her later years. Not only had she become enlightened in those last twenty years, but she had modeled for me and for everyone in my family that it is never too late to change or grow.

I think the most important thing I learned from watching Mom die is that her death was hers, not mine – just as her life had been hers and not mine.

Honor and privilege

It was a privilege to care for Isabel Emmott-Haller and Mable Clark. David and I were honored to be at the helm of their care. It is my sincere hope that their lives and the lives of all those whose stories are contained in this book have borne witness to two simple but profound truths: the aging ones in our families matter, even when they are frail, ill, and confused. They matter in their living, and even more, in their dying. And we can make a difference in their lives by accompanying them as they age. We can walk with them, talk with them, and be their voice when theirs is silent.

As we drove through the mountains in Colorado last week, David and I had one more conversation about the care of our mothers and the lessons that we have learned from the experience. I read him the last two chapters of this manuscript. We revisited our journey – beginning with how surprised we were that so many of our families' decisions fell to us. Yes, we are in the medical field, but we had lots of female siblings (the usual choice for caregivers in families) and lots of older siblings. And, then we realized that our experience is not unique: it is exactly what happens in all families. Yet many of us think that caring for Mom or Dad or Aunt Bessie or Uncle Tony will fall to someone else, not us.

The unavoidable outcome of this naïve thinking is that we are not ready to take on the role of caregiver or decision maker. David and I agreed that our advice to all family members is to assume that, indeed, it will be you who is asked. That way, you can keep part of your life available and open for this sacred work. And you will know, early on, that it will not be easy or quickly resolved. That's the honest depiction of what can and most likely will occur as your parents age.

The ultimate life lesson that David and I learned is surely important: there is an undeniable relationship between preparedness and a sense of no regrets. Get ready. You can do this. You can help your parents die with dignity and love.

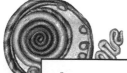

Lessons for Living without Regrets

- Aging itself is a type of grieving, a time of change, and change nearly always includes loss.

- One's emotional pendulum swings from celebrating memories to grieving a loved one's absence.

- How we love and respect our parents will influence how our children care for us in our time of aging.

- We can honor those who have gone before us even after their lives on earth have ended.

- There is an undeniable relationship between preparedness and a sense of no regrets.

CHAPTER 2

Beginning the Work
Exploring What Matters Most to Your Loved Ones

My husband, David, teases me about the books on my bedside table: *How We Die* by Sherwin Nuland: *Talking About Death Won't Kill You*, by Virginia Morris; *In Defiance of Death* by Ken Fisher; and my all-time favorite, Leo Tolstoy's *The Death of Ivan Ilyich*. I use these books and others in healthcare ethics courses. Tolstoy's eighteenth-century tale is always popular and forms the backdrop for a high school course called "Philosophy of Life – Philosophy of Death."

Tolstoy was obsessed with death and dying, but his character Ivan Ilyich never gave it a thought. Ivan was like every young, aspiring man of today. He worked hard to achieve the professional and social success that he believed would insure a perfect life. Then one day, he climbed a ladder to straighten the drapes (custom-made, no doubt) that workers had recently installed in the formal sitting room of his new house. He wanted the house and the drapes to be perfect when his wife and children arrived. Ivan fell off the ladder, however, and his life changed dramatically.

The fall had irreversible medical consequences. Henceforth Ivan lies helpless, writhing in pain, as friends blithely pursue the perfect job he can no longer fulfill. He is astonished and bitter. His friends do not ask for, or seem to miss, his company or his knowledge.

His family, too, carries on without him. They happily attend operas and other social events as he lies disabled and slowly dying.

Bereft, Ivan finds no relief. Not even his doctor tells him that death is coming. He screams in pain, and careful readers know that his pain is both physical and spiritual. His screams reveal his disappointment and great anger. He is angry at himself for believing that he could buy a perfect life and at society for its support of a life so void of depth and meaning.

My students are struck by two thoughts: how little Ivan communicates with his friends and family, and how easily his friends ignore his impending death and simply go about their daily lives. They often refer to a passage in the book in which Tolstoy says that Ivan's death evoked in his co-workers, the people he spent most of his time with, nothing more than "the usual feelings of relief that it was someone else, not they, who had died."

Tolstoy's tale suggests that it is natural for us to think that leading a productive life and striving for the best is sufficient to make us happy, or that life itself will protect us from unwanted events like accidents, ill health and, ultimately, death and dying. Ivan's experience forces us to question that assumption and to think about life as Tolstoy did, through the lens of death and dying: "Do we need to talk about what matters in life?" "What do we value in life?" "Are life and death related?" "Should we talk about death and, more specifically, should we talk openly about our own death?"

I end the course by asking each student to describe a "good death," the ultimate challenge for each of us.

When I put these questions to students, their initial response is hesitant, but soon they are talking openly about everything from the loss of their first pets to their feelings and fears about death and dying. Many students begin the session with sad and fearful stories, but over time, their stories are transformed in the telling and become life changing.

I end the course by asking each student to describe a "good death," the ultimate challenge for each of us. It is not an easy discussion for them. By the end of the course, however, most of the students can talk easily about what is important to them in life and what frightens them most about dying. They are on their way to developing a philosophy of life and death that I hope will guide and enrich their futures.

Thinking about death in the abstract is very frightening, the more so when it is our own death that we are contemplating. No wonder most people simply refuse to discuss it – or use humor or some other tactic to deflect the emotions it evokes. Only on rare occasions does death confront us in life, and its depiction in the movies is often surreal. After seeing the movie, *Million Dollar Baby*, one of my friends made me promise to shoot her if she ever got in Maggie's condition. "It's so inhuman and degrading to be dependent," another friend said recently.

> *It is not an easy discussion for them. By the end of the course, however, most of the students can talk easily about what is important to them in life and what frightens them most about dying.*

"If I ever become helpless, please just give me the bitter pill." Sometimes these comments are accompanied by grim humor and no serious response is expected. "Sure," I mutter, "no problem." But I know that this is a dishonest response.

My friends' requests are not based on real life, but on what happens in movies. In the *Million Dollar Baby*, Hilary Swank plays Maggie, an aspiring welter-weight, female boxer who asks her boxing coach, Frankie, played by Clint Eastwood, to end her life. Maggie wants relief from the miserable life she must endure after a boxing injury paralyzes her every limb and eventually requires the amputation of her leg. She can no longer do anything she formerly enjoyed. She cannot move or control her body, and she is totally dependent on a breathing machine. Frankie visits Maggie everyday and each time she pleads with Frankie: "Please kill me."

Frankie and Maggie are not just coach and player. They are more like father and daughter. In fact, Frankie nicknamed Maggie "Mo Chuisle," an Irish term for "my darling," "my blood," literally "my pulse." Frankie is so tormented by Maggie's condition and her relentless requests that he confesses his quandary to a priest and is quickly and emphatically told that euthanasia is a sin.

Talking about death and dying is the ultimate conversation stopper, and the request to just shoot me or give me the bitter pill is a futile effort to deny thinking about death.

Eventually, however, Frankie is unable to bear Maggie's suffering. He sees her trapped in a useless body that had once brought her release from a life of poverty and servitude to an uncaring family. He injects Maggie with epinephrine which causes her immediate death.

Sometimes I can hear the anguish my friends' comments mask, especially if they have recently experienced the long drawn-out death of a loved one. But I'm a nurse, and honestly, I really want to throw up my hands and shout at them. "Let's be more serious, my friends!" On the rare occasions that I insist on some honesty in the discussion, my friends think that I am being overly academic or professional. But in fact, they don't want to hear the truth. Talking about death and dying is the ultimate conversation stopper, and the request to just shoot me or give me the bitter pill is a futile effort to deny thinking about death. If we want to plan the part of our exit strategy that we can control, we must not be afraid to talk about what a decent and good death would be like for us personally.

Beware the tides

Terry Rosell, a friend and colleague of mine once gave a lecture on "The Good Death" in which he shared his personal sense of what a good death would look like. He said that he would consider a good death to be one that didn't include dying stupidly. I couldn't imagine what he meant by that. Then he described a trip that he and his family had taken to the coast.

They packed their lunches, towels, and cheerful attitudes and headed to the beach. Along the way they saw several warning signs posted about rip tides: "Beware of Undertow." Not wanting to disappoint his children or risk having them think he wasn't as cool as their middle-school friends, he entered the water. About ten minutes into the swim a wave caught him off guard and carried him under water. He was under water for so long that his chest almost burst. Sputtering and coughing, he searched for solid ground. It took a while. "I was very close to dying stupidly," he said. "I had ignored signs that were clearly posted."

If we want to plan the part of our exit strategy that we can control, we must not be afraid to talk about what a decent and good death would be like for us personally.

I had one of Oprah Winfrey's "aha" moments while listening to Terry's lecture. Everyone who is afraid to talk about death and ignores the opportunity to prepare for its coming is at risk of dying stupidly. The signs are all around us.

So back to my friends who, after seeing a film depicting unpleasant or unacceptable scenarios of death, request a quick exit for themselves. I need to cut them some slack. They probably never had a high school course on death and dying. In fact, many of them may never have thought about or discussed death with anyone.

As adults, we typically deny death, acknowledging it for the first time, only when our parents become frail or ill. And even then, we face it as though it were uncharted territory though we have all seen other deaths happen right before our eyes. Our memories are selective. It is easy, for example, to remember when Great-Aunt Bessie died in her sleep at age 83 but difficult to recall Uncle Ira's death, preceded as it was by ten long years of increasing frailty and memory loss.

Everyone who is afraid to talk about death and ignores the opportunity to prepare for its coming is at risk of dying stupidly. The signs are all around us.

Denying death sets us up to be buffeted by some very strong waves – the rip tides of caregiving and healthcare decision making that can drag even the best of us under water. Were there signs along the way alerting us to pay attention? Were there opportunities to talk about our values and wishes? Was there time to prepare ourselves to die other than stupidly?

A matter of timing

Very recently, while on a long car drive, I asked my husband David if he had spoken about death with either of his parents. He thought about the question for a long time before recalling that his dad, Dr. Ralph Emmott, had once talked to him about his older sister's brain injury. Karen was only sixteen when an anesthesia mishap occurred during a routine surgery at the very hospital where David's dad was doing his surgical residency. "It's been thirty years," he told David, "and the incident still haunts me. It is my greatest regret."

David said that his dad had told him this story when he and Isabel were visiting us to celebrate the birth of our third child. He used the story to tell David about Karen's disability, but also about life and death, fatherhood, and regrets. Years later, he asked David to serve as Karen's family guardian, a decision that could very well have resulted from this conversation.

I gave David a few minutes to collect himself before I pushed the topic of death a bit more. "What about your mother? Did you have any conversations with her about these matters?"

"No," he told me, "not before she got goofy." His mother, Isabel, had been the ultimate matriarch. She was breathtakingly beautiful, watched her waist line, and was always properly attired. More than that, she was an educated woman. It was Isabel Emmott who urged public schools in Oklahoma, to teach Latin. After all, she said, seven of the Emmott children will be educated in these schools. She drove six kids to swim practice at 5 A.M. hundreds of times, including one who became an All-American swimmer. Though she suffered a severe depression after "Karen's accident," she emerged from it and became the primary caregiver for her brain-damaged daughter for almost fifty years.

Denying death sets us up to be buffeted by some very strong waves – the rip tides of caregiving and healthcare decision making that can drag even the best of us under water.

How unfortunate, then, that no one ever asked her where she got her strength or how she felt about her parents' deaths, or what she had experienced when her children's father died and then her second husband, too. "Most of all," David said, "I regret not asking her to tell me about the kind of death she wanted for herself."

None of Isabel's children could have foreseen that in her early seventies, after the death of her second husband, she would retreat into a world of confusion and agitation. But David knew that it was not her dementia that had robbed him of the opportunity to have these conversations. In the many years before her dementia, he would have been a good listener, but they lived busy lives and the threads of denial intervened. "It was a timing thing," he said.

I reminded David that no one, not even doctors, know what the future holds or when it is the right time to talk about death. Then I told him about my grandmother. She didn't talk about her death until the last day of her 103 years! We both laughed and agreed that she had had all the luck! Indeed, on her final day, my grandmother managed to have a thoughtful, consoling conversation with her German physician, Dr. Ralph Heine.

Lucinda Angeline Clark, called "Grandma Clark," was a stern, God-fearing woman, the kind of woman people were a little afraid of. She wore dresses, heavy stockings, and black, laced-up, practical shoes every day. Using a push-mower, the kind that didn't take gas or self-propel, she touched up the lawn after the neighborhood kids had mowed for her, taken her money, and run off to the local candy store.

She raised nine children as a single mother after the early death of her "man," a postman who had delivered mail by horse in rural Oklahoma. Late in life, she fell and broke her hip and never returned to full independence. It became unsafe for her to live alone, but the staff she hired only stayed for short periods of time. They didn't please her and didn't do things the way she wanted them done. Goose-down mattresses weren't fluffed perfectly, rose bushes weren't trimmed correctly, and their cooking was impossible!

Eventually Grandma Clark moved to a small, family-owned nursing home in Elk City, Oklahoma, where she lived for several years. At some point after her last birthday, she quit eating and drinking. A few days without food and water and her heart rate increased. A nurse at the facility called Dr. Heine, who had been our family doctor for decades. It was Friday afternoon. Dr. Heine told the nurse not to bother her son, the reverend Joe Clark, but to place a temporary feeding tube through her nose and give her Ensure, a liquid source of calories. "I'll speak to the Reverend on Monday," he said.

Grandma would have nothing to do with this idea. When Renee, the licensed nurse, went into Grandma Clark's room to explain what she intended to do, Grandma shook her head, signaling a distinct "no." She pushed the nurse away. Renee had been part of the care team long enough to know that Grandma knew what she was doing. Indeed, Renee and her siblings had been among the neighborhood kids who had mowed Grandma Clark's lawn. She knew this woman and wanted to respect her wishes. She placed a second call to the doctor. He promised to come and chat with the older woman after his dinner.

Dr. Heine told us later that Grandma did most of the talking when he arrived. He checked her heart rate and blood pressure. He found changes associated with dehydration and heart failure. He encouraged her to eat or drink. She insisted that he drink some juice with her. Renee watched as the two drank apple juice from well-used, cracked coffee cups retrieved from the staff lounge. Dr. Heine sat with the aged woman and held her feeble hands.

Grandma sat up her final time and told him what her days were like. She couldn't hear the evangelists on the radio any more. Her six daughters had all died. Her three sons and their children were busy and rarely visited. She wanted to see her man, her husband again. It had been seventy years since she lost him. She wanted to meet her Lord. And, furthermore, she told Dr. Heine, earlier that week the staff had cut her long hair. The long braid that she had always worn neatly pinned into a low-set, distinguished bun was missing. She cried even as she assured him that she knew it was easier to wash her hair now and keep it clean.

Renee witnessed the doctor's quick journey to understanding and acceptance. Grandma Clark had reached the finish line, but she was not afraid. She had peace. She was in control. Renee told the family that Grandma Clark died about an hour after the doctor left. It was her choice. She had watched time ticking away. And finally, perhaps for the first time in their long doctor-patient relationship, she and Dr. Heine had talked about life and death.

Sit on your hands

Sister Rosemary Flanigan is one of the smartest people I know. She taught philosophy at a Jesuit university for years and after retiring, spent more than twenty years teaching ethics to community members and healthcare providers in Kansas and Missouri. She taught us how to help our patients and our loved ones make tough, end-of-life decisions.

Rosemary began many of her teaching sessions by shaking her finger at her audience and saying, "If I have a heart attack, right here, today, sit on your hands! Do you hear me? Sit on your hands! Do not attempt CPR." Rosemary, like Grandma Clark has lived fully and when it's time, she wants to die as she has lived – in control as much as possible.

A colleague with whom she shared an office was not sure he could comply with her wishes, but she made him promise to do so. "Okay, okay," he said. "I promise to do nothing if you have an untoward event."

"I didn't say, 'do nothing'," she replied tartly. "You may certainly hold my hand and pray with me." Sister Rosemary calls her approach "dying naturally."

Conversations about life and its ups and downs are cumbersome, but they are also great opportunities to explore what matters most to the people we love. We need to ask about their greatest joys and deepest sorrows. We need to find out where and how they want to die, and who they want to have with them at that time. We need to know what it is they still need to do before they can be at peace like Grandma Clark. These conversations will not be easy, but they will be our guide and solace when difficult decisions have to be made about a loved one's wishes and end of life.

There is no easy way to exit life when and how you choose. Instead we need to talk to our parents, our kids, our doctors and nurses. We should not die stupidly or allow others to do so.

There really is no bitter pill or coach like Frankie in real life, and you have no idea how hard it can be to die. Unless you live in the state of Oregon, Montana or Washington, have a terminal disease verified by two physicians, and are capable of taking a bottle of pain pills on your own, there is no easy way to exit life when and how you choose. Instead we need to talk to our parents, our kids, our doctors and nurses. We should not die stupidly or allow others to do so. It's a question of timing, of letting go of the threads of denial. And it's a challenge. Sages tell us that the longest journey begins with a single step. I urge you to begin the conversation, this hard work, now.

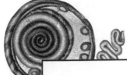

Lessons for Living without Regrets

- No one, not even doctors, know the manner or the time that we will die, but we don't have to die stupidly.

- Conversations help us focus on the part of dying that we can control.

- Sometimes we do most for a dying person just by being with them.

CHAPTER 3

Family Systems and Dynamics
A Two-edged Sword

Family dynamics are at the core of many, perhaps most, of the tough decisions adult children and their parents will face as they grow older. Our families of origin – our parents, brothers, and sisters, the people we grew up with – are the people we know best in life, so why has this chapter been so difficult to write?

Each of us is from an intimate, somewhat weird entity called a family, but when we try to describe our brothers and sisters and how they grew, we find ourselves enmeshed in memories and perhaps a bit tongue-tied; it's not an easy thing to live as a family. And, should anyone claim to have a flawless or highly functional family, he or she is in for a huge surprise when it comes to caring for aging parents. Even siblings whose early years were filled with peace and joy are not exempt. When it comes to joining hands and hearts together to care for aging parents, hurt feelings and sibling rivalries often recur, overtake events, and lead to chaos.

Let's face it: most families are a bit divided or have some interesting secrets to say the least. I know mine was. I was already thirty years-old, when I decided that I needed to reconnect with more of my siblings than the two who lived near me in the same city. At the same time, I began to question the rift between my mother and me. We hadn't been close since I was a teenager. For help, I turned to Murray Bowen's family systems theory. Dr. Bowen is a psychologist whose mental health focus is on the family unit rather than on the individual as Freud's had been. What I learned from his work was helpful, but it became really important to me when my parents and mother-in-law increased in age and began to experience ill health. It also helped inform my work on hospital ethics committees since so many ethics cases involve families in devastating situations and decisions.

Bowen believes that families are complex entities that are structured in patterns or systems that are passed down from generation to generation. He describes families as emotionally dynamic. Understanding family histories and how individual members interact emotionally with the system predicts and explains why family members act in various ways and why they react so emotionally when challenging situations arise. In this chapter I will again use my family experience and my willing friends' families to illustrate why and how this kind of thinking can ease the way for caregivers and families who find they must communicate across generational boundaries.

Defaulting to older, taller siblings

As one of ten children and a woman married to a man with six siblings, I hope I have picked up some street smarts to pass along about families – not mind you, as a family therapist, but only as it relates to how we make healthcare decisions. Family patterns of function and dysfunction will constrain or empower immediate caregivers and other family members. For example, many important decisions in my family of origin were only finalized when the older, taller siblings arrived. Four of the first five children born to my mother and father are much taller than the rest of us. So even if several of the younger (and shorter) siblings were on hand to address a serious family matter involving our parents, they had to stand meekly by until the taller, older siblings arrived!

We younger ones were quite capable of making decisions, but in all honesty, the community, our parents, and even we ourselves assumed that all important decisions would be made by the older siblings. They were the wise ones. Once, when our mother was in her seventies and living alone in a small town in Oklahoma, she fell and broke her hip. She was sent by ambulance to Oklahoma City for surgery.

Family patterns of function and dysfunction will constrain or empower immediate caregivers and other family members. For example, many important decisions in my family of origin were only finalized when the older, taller siblings arrived.

We all talked about her accident; we asked ourselves why and how it had happened, and whether she would be able to return home. I look back on this time with a smile on my face, partly because Mom recovered so well but also because even though she was very capable of participating in these conversations, they happened out in the hall, while she was flat on her back in the hospital room.

Our tall, elder siblings arrived and took over. They believed that Mother's "sleep aid" had caused her fall. "She shouldn't be taking all these things," they declared. Our beloved tall, taller, and tallest siblings took action. They decided to clean out the medicine cabinet of this very capable woman! As they shared this story with the rest of us, my younger sister and I sat in a corner of the room, laughing quietly with Mom, who had not taken any medication, or tripped on an area rug (another "tall" opinion). She had, in fact, fallen off the closed toilet seat when pulling on her stockings.

That is the way our family worked. Mother had a successful surgery, rehabilitated in a treatment center in Oklahoma City, and returned to a very clean medicine cabinet and a very cold bare bathroom floor. Families have certain ways of working, and my family is the perfect example of Bowen's assertion that family patterns are well-established. Decision-making patterns percolate over years, even decades. Individual members or subgroups in families function in familiar ways. In my family, a certain pecking order existed. After Mom and Dad divorced (in their seventies), this pecking order proved its effectiveness: the older siblings cared for Dad in Oklahoma, and Mom moved to Kansas City, where her three younger daughters lived and could take the lead in caring for her (when it proved necessary). But be assured. Even then, we always sought the opinions of our older (and taller) siblings.

Capable women vs. decisive men

Gender issues are another important dynamic in family patterns. Various cultures define male and female roles as inherently different, but in my experience even traditional and fiercely egalitarian American families develop behavioral patterns according to gender roles. It is often assumed that the oldest son will make family decisions. In my husband David's family, his older brother Cameron was the "go-to" guy for their family for many decades. He is not only the oldest male, but the first child to walk in his father's footsteps and become a physician.

Three very capable women are also part of the Emmott family mix. One of David's sisters was a master's prepared teacher, another was a nurse and mother, and still another raised three boys while working full time in the banking business. I asked David why he thought his sisters were rarely, if ever, included in family deliberations. He shared with me his father's belief that women were to be seen and not heard and told me that this belief had dominated the family's decision-making pattern as long as he could remember.

His father's sentiment, he said, was both implicit and explicit and rarely challenged.

Women were expected to be pretty and emotive, not rational and highly educated. Events in the family then bolstered this belief. After David's eldest sister Karen sustained a brain injury, his mother Isabel, who until then had been an equal partner in the family and active in the community, became immersed in Karen's care and had little time left to mentor the other women in the family. When David, like his older brother Cameron, chose medicine for a career, the pattern was already there. The three male physicians became the dominant family decision makers – as Cameron and David are to this day.

Life-long family resentments can simmer beneath the surface of this kind of gender imbalance. David and I recall how difficult it was for his family to decide where their mother should live during her last years of life. Because Isabel's oldest son Cameron is a physician on the west coast and her other physician son lives in the Midwest, family decisions had always been challenging. Most decisions were made smoothly, however, so long as their aging mother was able to remain safe and comfortable in her own beautiful home. And she did remain at home for many years even when she was receiving total care around the clock.

But such care is expensive. As her Alzheimer's progressed and her financial dependence increased, staying at home became less of an option. Decisions had to be made. Consensus among the Emmott brothers and sisters on this aspect of their mother's care was virtually impossible. David's sisters and younger brother had been disenfranchised for years, but on this matter, the siblings reached impasse after impasse. The long-established family pattern required women to stand back, express emotion, and allow men to be reasonable. But this time the pattern created a roadblock, and no unified decision was possible. The women wanted to continue Isabel's care in her home. Their feelings were sincere but impractical, and the desire to accommodate their sisters' sentiments created an intractable conflict for David and Cameron. It was difficult for any of the siblings to think beyond the impasse to what would really be best for Isabel.

Let the experts decide

Gender differences are not the only impediment to good decision making. Another erroneous assumption is that a family member's professional or social persona is a natural indicator of his or her fitness to make decisions for other family members. Some family members may be experts in legal, financial, and medical subjects. We treasure their advice, and frequently call on them for decisions requiring such knowledge. This informal give and take among family members is useful and unifying, but it also follows a pattern that soon assumes the form of an unwritten law. It seems logical to us to call on those same family members for decisions regarding an aging parent's healthcare and end-of-life planning.

Another erroneous assumption is that a family member's professional or social persona is a natural indicator of his or her fitness to make decisions for other family members.

The problem with this assumption arises when family members who have this expertise are also busier than other family members or live great distances from the community in which they grew up and where their parents still live. It is especially tough if these busy, distant experts are expected to be the family's primary decision maker, estate guardian, or healthcare proxy, and downright impossible if a single expert is expected to fulfill all three of these functions!

Legal and financial experts should not always hold the trump cards regarding life decisions. That is not only my opinion; it is also standard practice in many professional healthcare settings. Caring for aging or ill family members often requires multidimensional decisions and an interdisciplinary approach. In hospital settings, for example, we strive for expertise from many professionals or disciplines throughout the hospital. The clinical care team and the ethics committee want to hear from the cardiac surgeon who is the attending physician on a difficult case, but they also want to hear from the chaplain and home health nurse.

> *The voice of the person being cared for – the person for whom the decision is being made – is the voice that really must be heard.*

The same diversity of expertise and experience should be sought within families, and each decision maker should respect the others, regardless of their professional role within the family or society. I like to say that family decisions should begin as a broad discussion in search of consensus. Family members who represent homemaking, artistic or technical work, or labor in other fields than finance, law, and medicine deserve a voice in these discussions and have important insights and balance to offer their expert brothers and sisters.

Even as a member of a hospital ethics committee, I worked hard to bring the voice of nonhospital professionals to our decisions to provide balance and commonsense. On one such committee, a gas station owner joined our committee, and we learned from him how a regular guy feels about things like feeding tubes and breathing machines. For the three years he served on the hospital committee, he frequently reminded us of the Golden Rule. Not a bad reminder when making decisions about health and aging.

Notwithstanding the importance of every committee or family member, it remains true that the voice of the person being cared for – the person for whom the decision is being made – is the voice that really must be heard. If this person is an aging parent, then his or her perspective is what our deliberations must reflect. If they cannot speak for themselves, then we must learn by listening to each other and especially to the family member who best knows their stories, values, and predilections. Knowledge that comes from the whole family unit is primary and the guide to how the medical, legal, and financial aspects of care can be arranged.

Challenging the family dynamic

Ethics committees make recommendations in difficult cases in which medical staff and family can't reach agreements. Often the source of the disagreement or conflict involves family dynamics. Millie's story is a case in point. The clinical care team asked the ethics committee to help them resolve a conflict involving Millie and her two sons. Millie was eighty-three- years-old and very spry. Each Thursday she drove to the beauty parlor to have her hair styled before driving to square dance on Thursday evenings. Then one afternoon, her car was broadsided on a nearby highway as she was returning from her hair appointment. She was life-flighted to Kansas City. Even though she had a grown son, an artist, who lived with her, her other son, a dentist, served as her durable-power of attorney for healthcare. He was also guardian of the family estate, which included a small farm in rural Missouri.

Millie had exploratory surgery and no internal bleeding was found. She was not conscious but a CT scan of her head showed no bleeding. Over a period of ten days, Millie gradually regained consciousness but remained confused. She had trouble eating because of the confusion. The medical team explained to her sons that a feeding tube might extend her life, but that she was unlikely to recover the health she had enjoyed before the accident.

Her two sons had different lifestyles and different ideas about their mother's future. John the dentist was sure that his mother would not want a feeding tube and certain that she would not choose to live in a long-term care facility. Tim, on the other hand, said that he had lived with her a long time and since her CT scan had not discovered a brain injury, she would certainly recover. It would take time, but he had lots of time to spare for his mother.

Tensions arose between the brothers. As the committee listened to the two men, it was clear that John had been appointed by his mother because he was well-educated in the medical field. Over the years, Tim had been dependent on his mother financially and had struggled to find a stable profession. In truth, however, Tim had spent much more time with his mother, listening to her and understanding what was important to her. John had been absent from the small town for many years.

The ethics committee's role was to help John and Tim communicate their different evocations of their mother's wishes so that John's opinions as the healthcare proxy could be informed by Tim's current depictions of his mother's values and wishes. It was a challenging job because their division of labor and family roles had begun when they were young boys. The committee recommended that blending the two perspectives would allow for a trial period after which the feeding tube could be withdrawn if Millie did not improve. This solution might have been the best solution but trial periods only work when there is great cooperation between family and the medical teams. In Millie's case, you can probably guess who made the final decision. I wonder what they would say now, eight years later; and I wonder if they have any regrets.

Such conflicts may be easier to handle if we realize that although siblings originate in one family, as adult children, they begin new families, live in different and sometimes distant communities, and embrace varying values over time. And even those who remain in the community of their childhood may live in different social environments and income structures. No wonder their daily values and life goals diverge. An older sibling may live two thousand miles away from Mom and enjoy a high income stream while a younger sibling lives closer to Mom and works from pay check to pay check.

Another common family dynamic is the tendency to attempt to settle old family resentments through decisions about Mom and Dad. Individual family members become very stubborn. These behaviors are apparent throughout the final stages of caring for an aging parent and may continue even after he or she dies. Some families experience what appears to be a "vulture-like" syndrome in which relatives flock in to scope out possible financial benefits or scoop up "things" from their parents' homes when the time comes to downsize or move out of the family home. Family members recall Mom saying "I really want you to have this someday" and last minute attempts to rehash old grievances lead to conflict. Even though David and I don't like to talk about it, tensions got so high when we moved Isabel into assisted living that we were accused of stealing some of her art. Interesting, to say the very least.

I once heard a hospice nurse compare family members to seagulls. I asked her what she meant. You know, she said, "They tend to fly in at the last minute and crap all over everything."

Making Mom's and Dad's best interest the guiding force

The best advice I can give concerning family dynamics is this: begin by recognizing the interplay and tensions between family members and their accustomed roles. Identify and acknowledge the long-standing family patterns that operate just beneath the surface. Take those that work and leave the others behind. There is no neat and tidy way to tie a bow on these dynamics, and the last thing you want is to use your mother and father's aging years to rekindle family dysfunction and resentments. Use your parents' stories and values to guide your processes. Ask questions that continually guide the process back to what is in the best interest of the person you are caring for.

My siblings range in age from 83 to 51 years-old. This range in our ages is a blessing and a curse. The blessing is easily identified: lots of wisdom, life experiences, and perspectives. The tough part is that we not only vary in age but in values and priorities. When faced with healthcare decisions, some of us are so practical that we seem complacent while others pursue answers on the internet and want solutions from centers like the Mayo Clinic or M.D. Anderson. When faced with dilemmas regarding our parents' aging and ultimately, their dying, we had to constantly remind each other that Mom's and Dad's best interests were the guiding force, not our own values and often selfish wishes.

> *Use your parents' stories and values to guide your processes. Ask questions that continually guide the process back to what is in the best interest of the person you are caring for.*

Interestingly enough, a good example of these varying opinions, was evident when we discussed our mother Mable's funeral and burial choices. We were reared in a rural part of Oklahoma where the common practice after death is embalming, open-casket funerals and burial at one of the small country cemeteries where other family members were laid to rest. However, part of Mable's new found independence was to break that mold. She complained that open-casket funerals were downright weird and that country cemeteries were not maintained to her standards. She insisted that she be cremated and her ashes interred where there was little or no maintenance required.

The desire to be cremated was really outside-the-box thinking for a few of my siblings. Sure enough, even to the end, we were still discussing these options. When Mother lost consciousness during her dying process, one of my sisters asked me tearfully if we could have an open-casket funeral before mother was cremated. As hard as it was to tell my grieving sister otherwise, I told her that Mother's views would be strictly adhered to while she was living and always. Her wishes would be honored.

My sister, who lived near where we were raised, didn't get to visit Mom often, and it was hard for her to accept that Mother's directions were the trump cards in this case and not the traditional ways of our past. To ease her pain, I told my sister that we would call her often and take every advantage of telephone calls, email photographs, and other ways to help her be present to and witness Mother's dying and be at peace with Mother's decision.

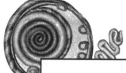

Lessons for Living without Regrets

- Knowing how individual members interact within the family system helps predict and explain how they will react in challenging situations.

- Caregiving decisions may be easier if we acknowledge that even though siblings have a single family of origin, as adult children, they begin new families, live in different and sometimes distant communities, and embrace diverse values over time.

- Knowledge from the whole family unit is important. In caregiving, all family members have important insights and balance to offer their expert brothers and sisters.

- The voice of the person being cared for – the person for whom decisions are being made – is the voice that must always be heard.

- Use the dynamics that work and leave the others behind.

CHAPTER 4

Choosing a Proxy Decision Maker
Who Will Be My Voice?

In the preceding chapters, we have discussed the need for thoughtful and ongoing conversations with our parents or other aging relatives about the values that give their lives meaning. And I have encouraged you to engage in an honest review of individual family systems. Painful moments may occur during these conversations. There may be family tensions to be tested and resolved, but it is rare for families who engage in these conversations not to gain courage in the face of illness and a greater understanding and acceptance of each other.

In this chapter, I will explore stories that will help you assist your parents as they seek to identify and empower a person or persons to be their advocate – their voice – when they are no longer able to speak for themselves. The choice of this advocate, usually referred to as a surrogate (substitute) or proxy decision maker is often the first formal step in the process called *advance care planning*, and it is imperative that the right person be identified and informed about his or her role and responsibilities.

This "appointment" or "delegation" involves more than simply asking someone to act in this role. At this time your parents will ask and empower someone who knows them well and who knows their values, desires and goals to step into their shoes. This person will be their proxy – their voice and advocate – when they are no longer able to make or communicate their own healthcare decisions. The documents used to appoint and instruct these proxies (your parents will each have a proxy and may or may not appoint the same person to act for them) can also be used to introduce these important persons to the doctors and other professional caregivers who will be involved in caring for your parents.

I encourage you to address this delicate issue with your parents sooner rather than later. My experiences as a nurse, ethicist, daughter, and friend have taught me how important it is to appoint the right proxy. Many times aging parents assume that the other spouse or the oldest son will take on this responsibility. But for many reasons, the assumed choice is not always the right choice. The right proxy will not only know your parent's values and desires; he or she will also have the strength of mind and heart to carry out those wishes when other family members might want to encourage something else. The presence of a strong advocate who knows their wishes is absolutely the best chance your parents have to avoid chaos and confusion and remain in charge of their important future healthcare decisions.

The right proxy will not only know your parent's values and desires; he or she will also have the strength of mind and heart to carry out those wishes when other family members might want to encourage something else.

Thinking and talking about issues surrounding substitute decision making touch on things that make us uncomfortable: aging, disease, and mortality. It's simply easier to rock on in life denying that these matters are already affecting our parents' lives and are looming in our future. A family in crisis needs a champion ready to go into action, and the person or persons who will be that champion must also be prepared and committed to the task.

Much of my career has focused on developing advance care planning tools and bringing public awareness to these matters. This focus allows me to see clearly not only how valuable the substitute decision maker is but also how difficult it is for families to take this first step in formalizing their plans.

Ideally, conversations about appointing a proxy should begin when both your parents are well enough to think clearly about what they want and about who would be their best advocate – that is, who among their family members and friends will know best how to stand in their shoes and keep the focus on what they want, even if it contradicts the proxy's deepest feelings. If, however, your parents are already experiencing a degree of frailty or ill health, these conversations should take place as soon as possible – on one of their good days when they are clear-headed and alert.

Your role at this time is to help your parents understand how important it is to choose the person who will speak for them when they are unable to make their own decisions. You can also help your parents and other family members know how this decision fits into the bigger picture.

Understanding the Durable Power of Attorney for Healthcare

Advance care planning is like a huge umbrella that covers all sorts of things like anticipating healthcare needs and making one's last will and testament. Your family will need a financial power of attorney or another legal instrument (form) to honor your parents' wishes regarding the management and disbursement of their financial assets. However, this book does not address the financial aspects of advance care planning. Our concern is limited to advance care planning related to your loved one's healthcare needs. Two questions suffice to govern this process. Ask your parents to consider how they would answer each of these questions: "What healthcare treatments do I want to receive or not receive when I am seriously ill?" and "Who will make my healthcare decisions when I cannot?"

These are distinct questions and there are different documents to help us record our preferences. The document answering the first question is called a medical or healthcare preferences directive and will be covered in a later chapter when I help you explore goals of care for your parents. The second document names the person your parent(s) have chosen to be their proxy – their Durable Power of Attorney for Healthcare Decisions. This document empowers the chosen proxy to speak for them, that is, to consent to, or refuse, any medical treatment for them (as directed in

Two questions suffice to govern this process: "What healthcare treatments do I want to receive or not receive when I am seriously ill?" and "Who will make my healthcare decisions when I cannot?"

the document). Some people refer to this person as their "agent" "surrogate decision maker" or "proxy." Others refer to the person named in this document simply as the "durable power of attorney" or DPOA. As you may have noticed from the previous paragraphs, I personally believe the term "proxy" is preferable.

The durable power of attorney for heathcare document becomes effective only if or when your parent or parents are no longer able to make or communicate their own decisions. A forerunner to this document was called a living will, but a living will was effective only when the person had been diagnosed as having a terminal illness. The DPOA, by contrast, enables the patient to have an advocate whenever he or she becomes incapacitated, and for as long as the incapacity lasts. It's important, therefore, to understand the concept of capacity, which is often confused with the concept of competency.

Recognizing incapacity

Many times, families, nurses, and doctors confuse capacity with competency. Competency is related more to the ability to reason and understand complicated ideas or perform a job of some type (for example, ability to pay one's bills, manage finances, or drive a car). Capacity is the ability to weigh value-based options and make decisions. What do I want for dinner? Do I want to have a chaplain visit? Should I have additional surgeries at my age?

When my mother was hospitalized with a broken hip, my older and taller siblings stood in the hall talking about what should happen to Mother when she returned home. That is, they assumed decision-making responsibilities for Mom because she was injured. They further assumed that poor judgment had led to her injury. (They wrongly thought she had taken a prescription to help her sleep). In fact, however, Mom was fully capable (or capacitated) at that time. That is, she was able to listen to alternative choices regarding her health and healthcare, weigh the risks

We should not usurp the role of decision maker before Mom or Dad is really incapacitated on the assumption that it makes healthcare decisions easier for healthcare providers and ourselves.

and benefits regarding those choices, and choose the treatment that was right for her. In other words, she was capable of deliberating and expressing her wishes and values. She did not need any of us to assume the role of healthcare decision maker for her at that time.

Families often assume that making decisions for those they care for and care about is their right and duty as part of compassionate caring. But preemptive decision making fails to recognize the dignity of each person. So long as a person has capacity, he or she has not only the right, but the duty, to make his or her own decisions. We should not usurp the role of decision maker before Mom or Dad is really incapacitated on the assumption that it makes healthcare decisions easier for healthcare providers and ourselves.

Thus, a mentor and good friend of mine in the field of healthcare ethics frequently says that healthcare providers and families think Mom and Dad are fully capacitated when they agree with the medical treatment being offered. But when, on the other hand, they say "no thanks" to suggested treatments, the family and doctors quickly assume that they have lost their ability to deliberate and need someone else to make their decisions. My mentor calls this the "nodding and bobbing" syndrome. As long as patients in hospitals and residents of nursing homes nod and bob, they are treated respectfully.

When my Dad was diagnosed with prostate cancer, his capacity was immediately questioned. He was, you will recall, a religious man who didn't prize medical care as an important resource for his well-being. Instead, he took a very passive approach to a cancer that his doctors considered very treatable. The doctor in his small town referred him to a university hospital in the state where I grew up and where my husband David did his initial training in surgery. The head of urology, who knew David, called him to express concerns that "Reverend Joe" might be losing it, that is, might be exhibiting early dementia or loss of capacity. His evidence was that Joe was making decisions on the conservative side of his treatment options.

David chuckled and told the department chair that his father-in-law had his own way of doing things and suggested that perhaps he ought to talk with me about how my dad was doing. I thought later it wasn't really *how my dad was* but *who he was* that influenced his decisions. His story shows how easy it is to be suspicious of decisions our aging parents make, and how easy it is to assume that they have lost their decision-making capacity when their choices are not what we want or when they do not insist that everything possible be done for them.

The truth is that my dad died as he had lived. He died in our old family home with hospice care. On the morning he died, he was found in his most comfortable chair, with his magnifying glass and Bible in his lap. Dad's life had always been challenging, and during his final months he was hearing and visually impaired. He could not manage his finances or drive. But he never lost his capacity to understand what was happening to him or who he was. He died in the same faith and courage that had supported him all his life.

Getting time on your side

When should you approach substitute decision making with your parents? The truth of the matter is that this choice should be made sooner rather than later. Time can be a precious commodity with aging loved ones. I remember when the initial episodes of agitation and forgetfulness began with David's mother Isabel. We were blindsided!

We had driven to the small town where she lived in Oklahoma to pick her up and drive on another hour to Tulsa, Oklahoma. We were on our way to attend a high school football game. Our son Cameron's Kansas City team was playing a Tulsa team on a Friday evening. We stopped at Isabel's home and, uncharacteristically, she wasn't ready to go. We had to help her get organized and choose a warm jacket. As we began the drive, David asked her what route was faster. She was literally dazed. She could not recall the fifty-five mile route from Bartlesville to Tulsa, a trip she had made hundreds of times over a period of thirty-five years. She not only couldn't remember but was agitated that we thought she should know it.

Over the course of the evening, she became confused about who was playing football. Was it her son Cameron or her grandson Cameron? John, Isabel's second husband, was alive at that time but he was in poor health and had never mentioned to us that Isabel was having periods of confusion and agitation. Now, however, the cat was out of the bag.

David and I knew after that weekend that Isabel's health was changing, and we were immediately inundated with questions. First, who would make decisions for Isabel when John was no longer able to make them for her? Isabel had assumed, as many aging women do, that her spouse would naturally fulfill these surrogate responsibilities. But John, like many spouses, became frail and eventually died before she did.

Your parents may hold this same belief or other assumptions about who should be their decision makers. For example, many people think the eldest son should be the decision maker even if this son lives miles from where he grew up and does not stay in touch with other family members. Your parents may believe that their appointed estate trustee or lawyer will make their healthcare decisions. Eliminating these types of mysteries and myths begins with informal conversations that can help clarify the truth and explore options.

Consider, again, David's mother Isabel. David and I knew that Isabel's neurological health was changing. We also knew that her husband's health was reaching a critical point. And, to complicate matters, David's adult sibling Karen was wholly dependent on Isabel because of her brain injury. Then, one day, another of David's sisters received a call from Isabel's hairdresser. She reported that Isabel had forgotten her appointment several times and had become uncharacteristically irate when she arrived on the wrong day. David scheduled a visit back to the town where he grew up. He took Isabel to a quiet place and had coffee with her. David asked her if she was aware of changes in her memory and in her mental status. "Yes," she whispered. She knew that she needed help. David asked her point blank, "Mom, who do you want to become your proxy?" She answered without hesitation, "You and Cameron."

It is an interesting fact that in the state of Oklahoma, the durable power of attorney for healthcare can be the same person as the guardian of the estate, so David and Cameron became co-guardians and co-proxy decision makers. Cameron was Isabel's guardian, but so was David, and David was geographically closer to Isabel than Cameron was. In all honesty, closeness can lead to a more realistic appreciation for what is going on at key moments of decisions.

> *Who would make decisions for Isabel when John was no longer able to make them for her? Isabel had assumed, as many aging women do, that her spouse would naturally fulfill these surrogate responsibilities.*

It was, for example, a difficult decision to determine where Isabel should live. Several of Isabel's children did not live nearby and work and family prevented frequent visits. David and I understood that they felt comforted knowing that their mother was still in her own home, surrounded by all the things she knew and loved. But as we watched her home and mental status deteriorate, it became evident to David that other options should be explored. I cannot count how many times this topic was broached, but it was not until the finances involved in her care and house maintenance preempted other concerns that the family could agree to make other arrangements for her safety and comfort. After much consultation, they agreed to place Isabel in an assisted living facility and hire extra care staff to insure her comfort and well-being.

Long-distance involvement in decisions, especially in a chronic co-guardian situation, can be taxing. There were times when feelings were hurt, misunderstandings occurred, and important decisions were delayed. At times, David would become weary and forget that his role was to make decisions in his mother's best interest – not to keep everyone in the Emmott family happy. David and Cameron, were co-guardians and co-agents for Isabel's healthcare decisions for almost ten years. That is a long time for two very busy physicians to communicate and collaborate especially when one is in the Midwest and the other on the west coast. It is also a long time to balance the roles of healthcare decision maker and shepherd of financial resources.

Knowing whom to appoint

So, how do we choose an appropriate surrogate? Consider, yet again, how Mable, my mother, chose David as her surrogate decision maker. She appointed him as her proxy even though she had ten children of her own, any one of which might have seemed a more logical choice. She said it wasn't a difficult choice. "I know I can get lots of good care in Oklahoma. I know I have good kids there, but I choose to live in Kansas City, not because I think there will be more things available to me as I grow older. I choose Kansas City because I know that when I need healthcare, David won't let stupid things be done to me. I am a simple woman. I want to die a simple death."

She went on to say, "You girls (she had seven daughters) will not be able to give up on me when the time comes. David will help you. He's really smart about these things." That's how my mother, a woman with ten children, opted to move away from many old friends and several "tall" people in her family, to a town where three of the shorter and younger kids were, and her really smart son-in-law.

As a physician, David was not only good at interpreting medical options for my mother and my family; he was also a genius at including Mom when he could. He also included me as a point-person for my siblings so that we always had good options for communication. He never over-ruled any of Mom's decisions, but always listened to us and integrated who my mother was into all final decisions.

At one point, when Mom fell and hit her head, David asked her if he could put a butterfly band-aid on her forehead, so that she wouldn't have to go through the trauma of being transported to the hospital. Watching how kind and sweet David was with her convinced all of us that her choice could not have been better! Yes, it is unusual for a healthcare proxy to be a physician, but whoever can make kind, compassionate considerations for our vulnerable, aging parents is the right proxy even if he or she is not the most closely related.

The responsibilities of the surrogate decision maker are typically transitional, ideally beginning as a partnership with parents while they are able to make their own decisions, then escalating to include many obligations. These duties, which may seem insurmountable at times, can include emergencies requiring a person to drop all other things in

> *Whoever can make kind, compassionate considerations for our vulnerable, aging parents is the right proxy even if he or she is not the most closely related.*

life. And one's service in this role may extend over a period of years or even decades – especially now that people are living well into their eighties and nineties. David and I, he as the proxy for my mother and I as his supporter, spent countless hours gathering information, meeting with home health providers, visiting long-term care facilities, communicating with multiple physicians, and conveying information to various interested parties, including family members who were sometimes hard to satisfy.

A very common turning point for surrogates has to do with parents and driving. Many of our friends ask us about this issue. And, we were not untouched by this decision either. Realistically, however, it is not the duty of the healthcare surrogate to make this decision, which is more about competency than capacity. Competency, remember, has to do with one's ability to understand complicated ideas and perform certain jobs or tasks. Examples of changes in competency are poor driving, not paying bills on time, and deviations in one's usual patterns of commitments, such as going to hair appointments or bridge or bingo on the wrong dates.

Changes in these areas serve as signals to families that parents may be struggling to maintain competency in these areas. Often these changes are marked by overt times of agitation and frustration, so that it may be best to discuss decisions about these matters – bill paying and driving safety – with the family attorney or your parents' primary physician. The proxy decision maker may be a helpful resource to the family in many areas, but his or her responsibility is only this: to make surrogate decisions regarding healthcare when and only when, your parents are unable to make these decisions on their own.

At the beginning of this chapter I noted that helping your parents choose a proxy decision maker is an important component of advance care planning. It follows naturally on the course you began when you engaged your parents in conversations about their life values and healthcare preferences. Having reviewed your family history – with, I hope, as much laughter as sighs – you probably have some ideas of your own and your parents no doubt have a fairly good idea of who they think should fulfill this role. Choosing a proxy confers a responsibility on the one chosen as well as an honor, and it doesn't mean that others in the family are not as smart, as beloved, or as important in caregiving. Ideally, having someone in this role will give each family member the freedom to do what he or she does best and to be present for your parents in his or her unique way.

Choosing a proxy confers a responsibility on the one chosen as well as an honor, and it doesn't mean that others in the family are not as smart, as beloved, or as important in caregiving.

As you continue your conversations and explore with your parents who the proxy should be, consider, again what it is you are asking the proxy to do. My mother's friends, and my younger friends, too, often tell me that what they fear most about aging is that they might lose control: "You know, lose my dignity, not be able to care for myself or to say what I want, or worse. I don't want to become a useless burden to any of my children." The proxy decision maker is there to ensure one's dignity, one's autonomy, one's right to be treated according to one's own wishes.

How does the proxy do it? First, he or she follows the oral or written instructions that the person appointing the proxy has previously provided. Note again, the importance of having these conversations, early, and often. This is the first model of proxy decision making.

Of course, when the instructions are given, the exact clinical circumstances that will require a decision will be unknown. If the instructions do not anticipate all the possibilities, the proxy decision maker may need to use a "best interests" model of decision making. In this second model, the proxy decision maker asks what is in the "best interests" of the patient. The decision to be made is simple: "Given what I know about my mother what is best for her?" The decision maker then gives his or her "best judgment" about a proposed medical treatment. This is an important model of substitute decision making, and it is particularly helpful when the appointed proxy has not been fully instructed about the person's values and wishes.

Recently, however, Daniel Sulmasy and Lois Snyder have proposed a third model of surrogate decision making. They refer to it as the substituted interests model. This model integrates the person's expressed wishes with the judgments of loved ones and physicians to determine what the person's wishes would be in this particular clinical situation. In this model, the central question the decision maker may be asked will be something like this: "What do you think your mother would tell us if she could speak for herself at this time?"

> *The proxy decision maker is there to ensure one's dignity, one's autonomy, one's right to be treated according to one's own wishes.*

I think this is a good model. Using my Dad's decision to approach his cancer care conservatively is a good example to help us think about the difference between the "best judgment" versus the "substituted interest" models. Let's say that the chief of urology at the teaching center who called David was correct in suspecting that Dad had some type of dementia. David would have called my older sister, Martha, and told her about the situation. As Dad's proxy for healthcare decisions, Martha could easily have chosen a more standard approach for Dad's cancer treatment. Using a "best interests or best judgment" approach to determine Dad's medical treatment, she could even have consented to a radical prostatectomy or radiation. Quite frankly, this decision would have been in keeping with a certain standard of care for his diagnosis. On the other hand, if Martha had asked herself what Dad's wishes would have been in this particular situation, her decision would have looked very similar to the course Dad actually chose.

A "substituted interest" model of surrogate decision making is a perfect fit for the formula that I support as I advocate for conversations with parents or aging relatives about what they value in life, encourage family system reviews, and urge the appointment of a substitute decision maker. The perfect proxy is someone emotionally in tune with your parents, capable of staying current with their evolving healthcare needs, including their mental status, and strong enough to accomplish their wishes. And, finally, a good proxy is able to communicate his or her reasoning to those caring for the patient and other family members.

If I have not yet convinced you of the importance of making a proxy appointment, consider what might happen to your parent if a durable power of attorney has not been made. It is roughly estimated that about 85 percent of aging Americans lack decisional capacity at the time of their death. In the absence of a duly appointed proxy, the state may decide who will make these decisions or may require the appointment of a guardian. Statutes vary from state to state and from court to court. Many states have enacted a "next-of-kin" statute which provides a prioritized list of surrogates. This list typically begins with the DPOA and includes family relatives (for example, spouse, adult child, sibling, adult grandchild) and ends with close friends or

> *The perfect proxy is someone emotionally in tune with your parents, capable of staying current with their evolving healthcare needs, including their mental status, and strong enough to accomplish their wishes.*

a state-appointed guardian. The goal is to find a "reasonable" person to make healthcare choices, but remember that the presumed surrogate, like the spouse or oldest son, is not always the best choice, and good candidates may be left out of the hierarchy altogether.

The choice of a proxy decision maker is one that only your parents can make. I urge you to encourage them not to leave it up to the state or to the courts. A court appointed guardian probably has the least chance of knowing your parents' wishes. (Even on the states' prioritized lists, the court appointed guardian is not favored.) That said, as the demographics of aging change and life spans increase, these statutes will be important for aging residents in long-term care facilities who may outlive many or all friends and family members.

Lessons for Living without Regrets

- The choice of a proxy decision maker is one that only your parents can make.

- Encourage your parents to choose a proxy and instruct him or her about their wishes and values as soon as possible – before they begin to experience ill health.

- Capacity is the ability to weigh value-based options and make decisions.

- Proxy appointments become effective when and only when a person no longer has the capacity to make or communicate his or her own decisions.

- The central question in the substituted interests model is "What would your mother tell us, if she could speak for herself?"

CHAPTER 5

Communication
Start with Being a Good Listener

At the best of times, communication is a difficult and challenging art, and never more so than when our topic concerns life and death and the difficulties we will encounter in caring for our loved ones as they age. No matter how often families resolve to have these conversations often and early, they still tend to occur later than we had planned and during difficult times. Acknowledging just how complex and overwhelming our task is in this regard has to be our starting point.

The truth is that achieving consistent and effective communication between our parents and their proxies and caregivers – and indeed with all family members and the larger community of friends and advisors who enrich our parents' lives – is absolutely essential. Without good communication, we cannot make decisions reflecting our parents' wishes and values nor can we secure medical care that respects their autonomy and dignity. Without good communication, our good intentions will not be enough to see us through the end of life with no regrets.

But first, a confession: The topic of communication and all that it entails is where our families' many warts reared their ugly heads. Maybe it was the size of our families or the dementia David's mother had or the length of time both our mothers survived while aging. We are not sure. But we are sure that missed opportunities for communication caused us many regrets. We were ill-prepared and frustrated on many occasions. As I recount some of the hiccups we experienced and the lessons that followed, I hope you will be better prepared. The lessons we learned involved three areas of communication: (1) learning how to define communication, (2) figuring out how to do it, and (3) knowing who should be included in the conversations.

In thinking about this chapter, I recalled my early training as a nurse. I was taught that communication consists of gathering information, relaying that information, listening and responding. I even recall being taught that nonverbal aspects of good communication are as important as information and that nurses should not be afraid to smile or shed tears, depending on the patient's need. I don't remember learning about other aspects of communication or having much time to explore even this definition in depth.

Proxies and caregivers generally need a great deal of practice or "seasoning" in communication, which they can only get from frequent exposure to their parents' lifestyle and values.

As you can imagine, such learning flew out the window as soon as I became a nurse. I knew from day one that communication would never be as simple as the one-on-one scenarios I had practiced as a student. Communication, I soon learned, involves entire families as well as multiple specialists who enter and leave the patient's care team as through a revolving door. I quickly resolved that my clinical and personal impressions were much less valuable than the more seasoned nurses' years of experience. This insight was confirmed and strengthened when I began working with aging patients and their families.

Just as family members who are well versed in legal and financial matters do not always make the best proxies (see chapter 3), so it is with highly skilled nurses. What all nurses need in addition to their professional expertise is something more akin to sympathy and knowledge – and this is what I saw among the seasoned nurses. Proxies and caregivers generally need a great deal of practice or "seasoning" in communication, which they can only get from frequent exposure to their parents' lifestyle and values and keen observation of how they respond to the myriad people they see each day.

A good proxy, like a well-seasoned nurse, will have many day-to-day experiences that will prepare him or her to meet multiple and sudden calls for communication – calls that will often come from many directions simultaneously and be accompanied by severe tension, grief, and loss.

Listening, time, and presence

A year ago, I took a course on listening, possibly the aspect of communication that most of us are least equipped to address. In the course, we were reminded that education, almost universally, includes reading, early practice in writing, and eventually, instruction in speaking. But rarely, if ever, are students taught to listen. I learned in this course that listening is not only a skill that must be learned; it is also a skill that reflects values. To be a good listener, the person listening must value the person they are listening to and be receptive to what that person is saying. The listener must slow down and be present to the person who is speaking. And most important, the listener must show respect. The notion of respect has huge implications for dealing with aging individuals, even our own parents. If we discount their credibility for whatever reasons – for example, personality, age, health, hearing status, or incontinence – our biases and prejudgments will have an unchecked effect on how we make decisions. In other words, the process of communication will be handicapped from the beginning.

Valerie Yancey, one of the finest nurses and lecturers I have ever known, uses many stories in her teaching and writing. One story that comes from her early years of nursing in an intensive care unit (ICU) illustrates an ethics of attentiveness. She was caring for a young patient who was seriously ill with end-stage liver disease. Her patient had tubes everywhere, in every orifice, and was receiving blood products and bleeding intermittently from his colon. As she began her shift, she busied herself about the room, measuring drainage tubes, calculating what fluids were left in the intravenous bags, and noting the stench of yet another bloody stool.

To be a good listener, the person listening must value the person they are listening to and be receptive to what that person is saying.

The patient was pale, and Valerie thought he was unconscious. His voice, she recalled, surprised her, when he suddenly asked, "What day is it?" She replied, "It's Thursday." He asked if he could go downstairs to a meeting that was scheduled to begin soon. She was shocked by his request and even a little annoyed. She continued her work, but he soon asked her again about the time.

"What meeting?" she asked. "Are you sure it's important that you go today?" He told her that his liver transplant support group met at the hospital on Thursday evenings. As she began cleaning his frail body, she told him that his condition was serious and even unstable. "I know that," he said, "but I need to go to the meeting. It gives me hope."

Only then did Valerie realize that listening to her patient was as important as attending to his body. As she maneuvered his wheelchair and multiple tubes and gadgets down the hall, she realized that the weekly transplant meetings, which gave him hope, did more for him than anything she could accomplish in the ICU. She was seeing only his disease, while the members of his support group continued to see him as a person.

Good healthcare proxies are attentive listeners. They hear when their aging parent is expressing his or her values and desires. Then as their parents' health declines and their capacity waxes and wanes, they can use the knowledge gained in the listening process to direct their parents' healthcare in accordance with their values and desires.

Time is the next important element in communication. We know from Valerie's ethics of attentiveness that listening takes time, and listening is only one element of communication. Communication also includes presence, and an effective proxy and other caregivers will not only spend many hours listening to their parents' wishes and values. They must also be available to help create appropriate times and settings in which their parents

The listener must slow down and be present to the person who is speaking. And most important, the listener must show respect.

will feel secure enough to share their innermost thoughts about how they have lived and how they want to die.

Talking about healthcare with aging parents has it challenges. Many times aging parents will cling steadfastly to their independence. They understand their children's desire to help, but they worry that such help also points to loss of control over their own lives. They dread having to reverse roles as happens in families when the formerly confident and competent parent becomes dependent on his or her adult child. So fiercely do they resist change that their hesitancy will look like sheer stubbornness. Often, however, they are simply confused and unable to partner effectively.

On many occasions when my sisters and I attempted to broach difficult decisions with our mother, she seemed totally uninterested. She would mostly talk about old times. We rolled our eyes through these long stories about the past, trying vainly to interrupt and refocus her attention. We were eager to get on with the tasks at hand. Considering choices and making decisions seemed much more important to us than hearing about past events.

We learned eventually that Mom's stories were not only important to her; they were also on point. She wanted to tell us stories that reflected on her diminishing autonomy. She wanted us to know that she had once been stronger and more in charge of her life. Once we acknowledged this need and helped create a climate of reverence, we could get to the heart of the matter. Efficient use of time took on a new meaning. Communication with Mom did not take place when people were rushed or preoccupied.

David's mother, Isabel, presented a different, no less challenging problem in communication. When she told us she planned to come to Kansas City for her grandson's graduation, we were concerned. We knew that she had dementia, though it was still in an early stage. She planned to drive, she told us, from her home in Oklahoma. Wary about her trip, we talked several times and devised alternative plans, but she insisted she would be fine. After many failed attempts to persuade her otherwise, she began the trip, making it without mishap, almost to Kansas City. Then the call came in from the highway patrol. She had been driving very fast and lost her way. We went south to meet her and a Kansas City police officer and David drove her and the dog back to our house.

David was on call that weekend, so I had to juggle a graduation party that included my extended family and both our aging mothers. I had to oversee three teens' activities *and* barter with Isabel about her dog's toilet habits. (Jack was a Bichon and Isabel went nowhere without him.)

At the time, I felt like David and I were teetering on the edge of a cliff, ungracefully trying to balance the impossible. In retrospect, I learned a valuable lesson in communication that crazy weekend. Thankfully, I asked our beautiful teenage daughters to help me out. Maggie and Libby sat with their nanny, listened to her stories about the past, and convinced her to let them take Jack outside from time to time. As I witnessed my daughters respecting their grandmother, I knew that David and I were finally learning how to be the adult children of aging parents.

> *Perfection and peace are not the goals of communication. Being true to the persons we are caring for, respecting them, and staying connected is what counts.*

I also learned another valuable lesson that weekend. Perfection and peace are not the goals of communication. Being true to the persons we are caring for, respecting them, and staying connected is what counts. What seemed like petulance on Isabel's part – the almost willful endangerment of herself and others on the highway and insisting on having the dog with her despite the inconvenience to us – was really her way of insisting on and battling for her integrity. She had been and would always be, even with dementia, an amazing matriarch.

Obstacles to communication

Aging can be accompanied by weakness and dependency, which fuel fear. David and I saw that happening to our mothers. Time after time, my mother would avoid answering questions from her healthcare providers or family members or she would answer in abrupt and curt ways. For example, unknown to us, my mother refused to drink adequate amounts of water. She had incontinence and correlated drinking fluids with her bladder problem. She would then become dizzy and confused – suffering symptoms similar to dementia or mild strokes. Efforts to communicate with her about this topic brought on a "none of your business" attitude that appeared to be plain stubbornness. At first, there were frequent trips to the hospital to find the cause of her symptoms – even a brain scan on one occasion. Later, we knew enough to request a urine analysis but decline a trip to the hospital. As she refused to make adjustments in her habits to fend off the infections, my sisters and I had to learn not to panic.

Communicating with Mom on the topic was so cumbersome that our responses had to change, not Mom's communication style or hydration habits. Even though my sisters and I were not the designated proxy, we were constantly at her side and served as her advocate. We communicated with David, her proxy. We soon learned that these early communication barriers in chronic matters such as Mable's

Communicating with Mom on the topic was so cumbersome that our responses had to change.

urinary tract infections and Isabel's early dementia and confusion, were preparing us for the more difficult areas of communication that were still to come.

I know now that what David and I were really learning in those early conversations was the underlying emotional aspect of communication, which was certainly not something we learned in medical or nursing school. It isn't just the words spoken or heard that make a conversation meaningful, but the desire for respect and trust that each one offers to the other.

Especially when things are going well for us, reticence, even a stoic refusal to talk about anything related to the end of life, is another obstacle that can threaten our ability to communicate with our parents. I hear frequently from my peers and colleagues that Mom and Dad answer all questions about their future healthcare wishes with comments similar to these: "You don't need to worry, we have everything taken care of" or "Mr. Smith, our lawyer, has everything in writing." End of discussion.

It isn't just the words spoken or heard that make a conversation meaningful, but the desire for respect and trust that each one offers to the other.

There are, of course, reasons for this reticence. Many parents, perhaps especially fathers, think that professional planning can shield their children and heirs from disagreements and grief. The adult children of aging parents may also be reticent. They may be uncomfortable talking about their parents' ill health or declining competency, so they, too, let the subject drop. Or they may decline to pursue the subject because they are hurt or offended to think that their parents assume they are only interested in how the estate will be settled. It is usually the case, however, that neither of these assumptions is true.

Too often, my friends discover that although financial and legal decisions involved in estate planning have indeed been completed, their parents have not discussed their values with anyone or documented their healthcare wishes. Where they want to live, how much medical intervention they want, and who they want to be with them in their last days has never been discussed. Conversations about these matters must be pursued and continued even when healthcare proxies and medical directives have been introduced and decisions made and documented.

An inclusive loop

Communication is an ever widening circle. It may begin in the immediate family as you and your parents consider whom they want to appoint as their proxy decision maker, but it continues in a more inclusive manner once that appointment has been made. I recommend that copies of all advance care planning materials be given to as many people as you can imagine. A short list would include at least your parents' living siblings and closest friends, all their children (that is, you and your siblings), and the physicians and other health professionals involved in their care. A more inclusive list would also include any attorneys and religious or spiritual advisors who are part of your parents' larger community. Sometimes a neighbor may be the very person to share your concern.

Think about the people whom your parents love and rely on for help. For example, David's mother had a psychiatrist on her team. She was the person who prescribed Isabel's anti-dementia medication. Later, when David and his brother chose to discontinue these medications, they realized that the psychiatrist hadn't a clue that Isabel wouldn't want heroic measures taken if or when she was in the final stages of Alzheimer's/dementia. Here was a person who definitely needed to know Isabel's wishes and the existence of her healthcare directive.

Don't be afraid to draw a wide circle. I recall a co-worker of mine who was an attorney and specialist in advance care planning. I always chuckled when he gave talks about aging, serious illnesses and advance care planning, knowing how he would end each presentation. Sure enough, no matter how small or large the audience, he concluded each talk by passing out copies of his Healthcare Directive and Durable Power of Attorney for Healthcare documents. You cannot make and distribute too many copies, he would say. The point of the documents, as of communication generally, is to make your wishes known.

Tools and tactics

Communication with your aging parents is important, but equally important to being an effective proxy is the ability to communicate your parents' preferences and values to others. An entire book could be written on this topic alone. I acknowledge that David and I are from unusually large families. He has six siblings and I had nine, though two of my older brothers died before my mother. Obviously, exchanging information, listening, and responding to everyone in families as large as ours is a huge undertaking. But the inherent job of the proxy is to be your Mom's or Dad's voice, and faithfulness to this task is essential to good communication. It is also the value that can help you be clear about your motives when communicating with family members and loved ones and this clarity is of great value regardless of your family size.

Again, I recall the huge barriers that David and I met when it was necessary to decide whether Isabel was safe at home or needed another place to live. Conversation after conversation occurred with and among his brothers and sisters about the risks and benefits associated with Isabel's placement. Should she remain in her home or move? And if she moved, should it be to an assisted living facility in their hometown or to a place near us in Kansas City? In the early years of communicating with his siblings about this issue, David's intention was to get their input. In later years, he resolved not to seek input but simply to inform them of decisions that he and Cameron would make based on Isabel's wishes or best interests.

A saying David and I frequently use when playing golf is "over-analysis leads to paralysis." This adage was certainly true when talking with his siblings about his mother. As his intentions changed from searching for consensus to giving information, he endured fewer long and tense phone conversations and wrote more informative emails, copied to all his siblings. But most important, Isabel's daily care improved dramatically.

I used emails to communicate with my large list of siblings. Several family members did not use emails, so I asked specific siblings to share the task of keeping them informed. I used emails and phone texts to share up-to-date photos of our mother. The photos were not only intimate; they also conveyed accurate and current depictions of her health status. Photos ranged from Mom enjoying an ice cream cone on her birthday to pictures taken when she was seriously ill. Indeed, we continued taking pictures until she died. I received many thank you notes for these communications – especially from those who lived too far away to visit her often.

Emails proved to be particularly effective when Mother became a hospice patient because the hospice organization also used emails extensively. Early in our partnership with them, I received emails regarding, for example, Mother's wheelchair size (too large, caused slumping) and her bed mattress. By using email, I did not have to rush to meetings with a member of the team. Instead, the team assessed each situation as it occurred and emailed me their suggestions and requests. They even emailed us regarding fees and reimbursable amounts. I in turn forwarded these emails to other family members to get their input. Then David and I would talk in the evening and make a decision.

As his intentions changed from searching for consensus to giving information, he endured fewer long and tense phone conversations and wrote more informative emails, copied to all his siblings ... Isabel's daily care improved dramatically.

In Mother's later stages with hospice, I got a weekly email from a nurse regarding Mother's health status and frequent emails from the hospice aide about her daily activities such as eating and walking. I cannot tell you how helpful and informative these emails were. I frequently forwarded them to family members with a note attached from me to help them understand how she was doing.

My sisters who lived near us were included in mother's care. My older sister Mary is a retired hair-dresser and salon owner. She assumed responsibility to assess and provide for Mother's hygiene and to keep us informed on this issue. It may sound trivial, but hygiene is an important part of caring for aging parents. When it goes well, their appearance, skin integrity, and general health are better. The assisted living facility and later the nursing home knew Mary's role and always addressed her concerns. She also let them know when she would need the salon. She herself cut and colored Mother's hair for many of her last years.

My younger sister Cinda worked as a paralegal for many years. She was Mother's guardian for all financial and legal matters. She communicated with the facilities where Mother lived and with us about reimbursement and long-term care compliance issues, such as hours of care, fall prevention, and, most important, Mom's daily activities. Cinda worked hand-in-hand with social workers and even a state ombudsman, which saved David and me hours of headaches. Mary and Cinda's involvement comforted Mom and allowed us to focus our time on communicating Mother's healthcare needs to the medical director and director of nursing.

The magnitude of communicating with healthcare team members is extensive. The chronicity or routine of healthcare issues with aging parents is inescapable, constant, and peppered throughout with fits and spurts of acute healthcare decisions. Healthcare providers are generally much better at monologues than dialogues, which makes the role of proxy or patient advocate more difficult. Knowing who to talk to and realizing that part of your role is to not let those in charge get away with bad communication is more than helpful – it's a prerequisite.

Research studies indicate that physicians nearly always interrupt patients and family members after listening to them for only twelve seconds. As a nurse, patient, and concerned family member, I believe that this finding is accurate. Residents in training and physicians also quite often resort to medical jargon when they speak. But jargon leads to misinterpretations and, ultimately, to misunderstood diagnoses and prognoses (that is, to a misunderstanding of one's disease and how it will progress).

Several years ago, the bioethics center where I worked hosted the family of Nancy Beth Cruzan at a seminar in Kansas City. You may recall that the Cruzan family battled long and hard with the Missouri and U.S. Supreme Courts for permission to remove Nancy's feeding tube after she was diagnosed to be in a permanent vegetative state, the result of a brain injury she had suffered in an automobile accident.

When Nancy was first admitted to a hospital in southern Missouri after her car accident, her medical team told her family that she had suffered prolonged anoxia. "We can only wait and see," they said. But one of her physicians also said that he was "deeply concerned about her anoxia."

Healthcare providers are generally much better at monologues than dialogues, which makes the role of proxy or patient advocate more difficult.

As her older sister retold the story she said, "We were deeply concerned about her anoxia, too. We just didn't know what anoxia was." Family members need to insist that medical professionals clarify medical terms and use plain English or descriptive terms to make medical situations clear to nonmedical but loving and smart people. As proxies or other advocates, we must be prepared to overcome such barriers to communication as constant interruptions or the use of medical jargon.

Follow the path of authority

Another important lesson that David and I learned was to find out as soon as possible who holds the decision-making authority in particular areas. For example, as Isabel's dementia escalated, she began falling frequently. Her falls resulted in hours, sometimes days, of angst, and many trips to the hospital for head scans, stitches for cuts, and much general concern about Isabel's well-being. She lived in an assisted living facility three hours from Kansas City. David had hired additional staff to assist his mother during the day – specifically, to help her bathe, dress, and eat her meals. This aide suggested that Isabel wear a helmet, similar to those that young children with head problems wear. David agreed, but days went by, and nothing was done. The aide was not employed by the facility and consequently lacked authority to make suggestions. Finally, after another incident, David spoke to the facility's director of nursing who obtained an order for the helmet from the medical director. The helmet was quickly obtained.

Knowing which primary care physician had privileges at the facilities where our mothers resided was an important step in streamlining communication. If no primary physician was on staff, who was the medical director, how often did he or she visit, and how could we reach them? And who were the directors of nursing, social work, and activities? It may sound time consuming, but getting this information is essential for proxies and other caregivers. You will also need to know when specialists are involved and how you can communicate effectively with them regarding treatment decisions. Two important decisions regarding Isabel's care were made only after David's brother Cameron (he and David shared Isabel's proxy for healthcare), discovered who prescribed her anti-dementia drugs, who could write orders to discontinue them, and who would carry out David and Cameron's decision to refuse ambulance trips to the local hospital every time Isabel bumped her head.

I will talk about their rationale for these decisions in the chapter on goals of care. Here I simply want to note that side conversations and phone calls with staff accomplished nothing until David and Cameron finally reached the person in authority. This lesson became invaluable to my family when we had to address our mother's treatments only a few years later.

Your communication with members of the healthcare team will change as your parents age and as their prognoses change. Usually communication will begin with in-home assistants and primary care doctors, and it may ebb and flow as your parents' wellness and illness patterns change. Acute situations may involve speaking with emergency room doctors. David and I spent much time speaking to Isabel's dentist because her dementia influenced her nutritional status which subsequently affected her teeth. In my mother's case, we communicated frequently with social workers as we strived to learn what benefits, including dentures and hearing aids, were or were not covered under Medicare.

Some of the most important information you will receive about your loved ones' status will come through those who are least empowered. I am referring to home health aides and certified nurse assistants, hair dressers, housekeepers, and even neighbors. Many times, they spend more time with your parents than members of the healthcare team. They often have great suggestions for changing or strengthening healthcare provisions, including dietary matters and safety. Don't discount the voice of anyone who has a true interest in the well-being of your parent.

David and I were both blessed and cursed with the obligations that come with large families. At times during the final years of our mothers' lives, it felt like we were Sisyphus, the ancient Greek condemned to roll a large rock uphill forever. We would resolve one area of communication and see light at the end of the tunnel, only to face another storm. But, by learning whom we should approach and how, and by reflecting on and adjusting our own motives and goals for communication, we were able to accomplish long periods of solidarity and unity. Perhaps Sisyphus couldn't be helped, but David and I learned that the rock is much easier to roll up the hill when others are pushing, too.

Lastly, I recall communicating with my mother during her last year. By then, Mom was ninety-five. Her biological body was worn out, and even though she never really gave in, she gave up a lot. Always an avid reader, she quit reading after a series of small strokes. Always a music lover, especially of old-fashioned country music and hymns, she gave up music when the onset of deafness made listening almost impossible. And although a great cook and lover of southern-style foods, she barely ate enough in her last months to keep a bird alive.

Some of the most important information you will receive about your loved ones' status will come through those who are least empowered. I am referring to home health aides and certified nurse assistants, hair dressers, housekeepers, and even neighbors.

Nevertheless, Mother loved to sit on a small sofa in the front atrium near her room at Sharon Lane Nursing Home in Merriam, Kansas. It was surrounded by windows, a large plant terrarium, and a hanging bird cage with a couple of brightly colored, constantly chirping birds. There were stacks of outdated magazines and daily newspapers on a table near the chair in which she sat for hours each day. Frequently when I visited, she would notice me and smile but didn't really say much. Eventually I would pick up a *Good Housekeeping* magazine and sit beside her, slowly turning the pages.

If I happened to see a photo of a lemon cake or a darling little baby, I would comment. She would smile as stories from long ago came back to her. "Remember when I made your favorite cake for your birthday and hid it in the kitchen cupboard? Your younger brother pointed it out the minute you got off the school bus!" She would smile and her blue eyes would twinkle merrily.

Other days, when the weather was nice, I would beg her to go for a car ride. She was always reluctant. "Let's just get in the car," I would say, "and if you don't feel well, we can just sit there." She would agree to the hard task of getting to the car. We would place her walker in the back seat and take off. Soon she would begin to notice blooms on the trees, cars passing by, and she would want to ride around a bit. There were times, however, when we just sat in the car. I would find a country music station and crank up the volume. She would smile, tap her toes, and on rare occasions, hum along.

Eventually I would pick up a Good Housekeeping *magazine and sit beside her, slowly turning the pages. If I happened to see a photo of a lemon cake or a darling little baby, I would comment. She would smile as stories from long ago came back to her.*

On the days we took drives, she looked out the window and asked questions about trees and flowers, large office buildings, and parking lots with hundreds of cars. "Where did all those cars come from?" "What kind of tree is that?" "I love Kansas City. It is so beautiful here." On many occasions I would park the car at an ice cream or yogurt store and run in and get cones for us. She loved strawberry ice cream. I would lick the drips falling from her ice cream cone just as she had licked mine when I was a child. We would get the giggles.

In her last year, most of our visits were like this. We didn't do much talking on these occasions because words no longer seemed so important. We weren't thinking about the past or the future; we were just together, enjoying the moment.

Communication with and about our aging parents is hard work, but the gain is no regrets. In some cases, the person changed by the experience will be the proxies (as David and I were changed); sometimes it will be the other caregivers, other family members, who are affected (as Mary and Cinda and all our siblings were changed); and sometimes it will be aging parents who get to hold onto their independence (as Mom and Isabel did). And yes, I can't resist noting: sometimes the entire medical team will learn how to redirect its recommendations to better reflect the wishes of their patients, our parents.

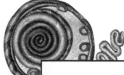

Lessons for Living without Regrets

- Resolve to have clarifying conversations early and often.

- Good communicators are active, attentive listeners who can help create times and places for sharing stories that reflect your parents' innermost thoughts.

- Perfection and peace are not the primary goals of communication.

- Communication needs will escalate as your parents experience diminishing health or increasing frailty.

- Proxies will want to develop and practice an inclusive model of communication with other caregivers and family members.

CHAPTER 6

Goals of Care
The Key to Asking the Right Questions

David and I discovered that a quintessential question kept recurring on our journeys with our moms. We found ourselves intermittently asking "What do I really hope for regarding Mother's care?" We used this question as a way to measure what we *should or shouldn't do*. Notice I do not say what we *could or couldn't do* for them. The difference between what we could do and what we should do is the essence of the lessons we learned and the key to establishing goals of care for your loved one. There are many things that *could* be done, but perhaps not everything *should* be done. The key to making decisions for your aging parents when they can no longer make decisions for themselves or each other is to ask yourself what should be done based on their preferences and on your hopes for them.

An encounter we had with a close friend is a perfect example of how a careful consideration of goals of care can help you make decisions with or for your parents when they are seriously ill or dying. In this case, the aging father was able to determine for himself what his goals of care should be.

Last summer, as David and I were driving back from a golf tournament in Tulsa, Oklahoma, we decided to stop over in Bartlesville, Oklahoma, to visit a long-time family friend, Big John Hoyt. We knew we would be saying our final farewell to Big John.

He suffered from chronic lung disease and had recently caught an infection that appeared to be the last straw for his tired body.

Big John was not big in stature, but in personality, he was a giant. He ran a large family company in which several, if not all four, of his children had worked at one time or another. He was the kind of man who balanced the "work hard-play hard" philosophy of life as well as any one I have ever known. He loved golf, his friends, his house in Michigan, including an immaculately kept 1960 Chris Craft boat, and not least his beautiful wife Gretchen, his grown son Johnny, three beautiful daughters, three grandchildren, and one great grandchild. Big John also loved a cocktail or two (or three) and playing cards. He smoked many a cigarette as he worked and as he played.

> *The key to making decisions for your aging parents when they can no longer make decisions for themselves or each other is to ask yourself what should be done based on their preferences and on your hopes for them.*

Over the thirty-seven years I knew the Hoyts, I never visited their home or family that I wasn't lovingly reminded that David really should have married one of the Hoyt girls. The tradition began when David and I were dating and visited his home town for our first Christmas together. During a Christmas party at the Hoyt home, I met the grandmother, Mrs. Freeburg. As she stood at the bar, tended by a family friend who also happened to be the local Episcopalian priest, she looked at me with kindness and some severity. "David Emmott can bring all the young girls he wants to home for the holidays," she said. "But he will marry one of my granddaughters." Father Evans told me later that he knew I was a keeper when I looked at her and said, "Really? I wonder which one.

I like all three of them." Over the next four decades, the only thing that changed is that I didn't just like the three girls. I loved them and the entire Hoyt clan.

Last summer, however, John and Gretchen's home had a somber air. Their son, John, and his wife Jen were there. Big John sat in reclining chair with oxygen delivered through nasal prongs from a tube that stretched from the master bedroom to the family room. He was struggling to breathe. Someone whispered that he had just finished a breathing treatment and needed time to recover from it. I sat down on the fireplace hearth. I could tell that all the guests, including my physician spouse, were terribly uncomfortable. There was not only a visible physical distance between them and John, but also the psychic distance that individuals establish in the presence of a person fighting for his life.

Weighing the options

After a few minutes, John wobbled over to the hearth and sat beside me. He thought sitting up straighter would help him breath better. I'm a nurse. I don't hold back. I hugged him. "This is no way to live," he said. I agreed with him. "You're right. When do you see the doctor again?" As we talked, I learned that he was on aggressive antibiotics and on the highest oxygen level that can be safely used at home. He was to see one of his doctors the following Monday.

I explained that hospice wasn't giving up anything that could really be treated at this time, and it would give him and his family control of his symptoms in their home setting.

I asked him if he had considered hospice care. He said that he wasn't ready to give up. I explained to him that what he needed most was to control the anxiety related to his fight for air. I explained that hospice wasn't giving up anything that could really be treated at this time, and it would give him and his family control of his symptoms in their home setting. We talked about things that addressed the quality of his life, such as his ability to eat, sleep, and even talk. He talked about the panic he felt as he fought for air. After our conversation, I knew he felt better. Maybe his treatment had taken effect or maybe he had a plan. I wasn't sure.

The next week I received this email from his daughter-in-law. She wrote:

> Just wanted to give you a big THANK YOU for your visit on Saturday - I learned A LOT from you!!!!!!!!!!! At the Dr. visit today the Dr. suggested hospice. John Sr. kind of shut down at that point and didn't hear anything else. However, when hospice showed up later at their home he realized, as you had said, [that it] is not a give up. They are going to continue to treat his condition but also focus more on his comfort level. He will have morphine available, at his discretion, to assist in breathing when HE says HE needs it. They also gave guidance in his daily routine. He was already much calmer when they left than when they showed up. Everything made sense to him and as you emphasized he is in control. I think everyone will sleep better tonight and that John Sr. will have a different attitude/outlook tomorrow. You planted the seed and it was reinforced today - with deepest gratitude, we thank you for this. . . .

I knew when I read the email that the conversation John and I had in front of the fireplace had helped him explore what he really needed from modern healthcare. It prepared him to partner with the doctor and figure out what he *should* do, instead of what he *could* do. Big John died a few weeks later. I heard he rallied before he died, even requested a couple of his favorite drinks, "Jack and water." He died painlessly and very much in control.

Big John had what I have come to think of as a good death. He did not want to lose control of his life. He wanted to be comfortable and to die at home. He didn't want to suffer because he knew that if he did, his family would also suffer. Control and comfort in his own home were his goals of care for his final days, and hospice care provided both of these.

Introducing a quality of life model

I have to be cautious when talking about how we die in America as I can become a lecturer and not the helper that I intend to be for you as you read this book. The sad reality, however, is that rarely do seriously ill and dying persons in our country, especially those who are advanced in age, die as Big John did. Roughly 75 percent of Americans, according to the Center for Disease Control, choose to die at home as John did. Yet, only 33 percent do. The other 66 percent die in nursing homes, rehabilitation facilities, or hospitals. I can live with some of that. Both David's mother and mine died in long-term care settings. But more important than where they died is how they died. The "how" one dies is framed by asking and answering questions related to their goals of care.

More important than where they died is how they died. The "how" one dies is framed by asking and answering questions related to their goals of care.

Dr. Betty Ferrell, a nurse researcher at City of Hope outside Los Angeles, is a close friend and colleague of mine. For the last decade, she has trained nurses in all areas of healthcare how to assist patients and their families to choose and receive good care at the end of life. The model she designed and proposed is holistic. It considers not only the physical aspects of well-being, but also the social, spiritual, and psychological dimensions of well-being. It leaves no stone unturned. Ferrell's model is referred to as a quality of life model, and she implores all nurses to use it as they work with dying patients and their families. Her rationale is that patients (our family members) are living while they are dying. Therefore, all decisions, especially those at the very end of life should be considered life decisions, not simply as one-dimensional medical or physical decisions.

David and I agree. When deciding what was best for his mother, we learned the hard way that if one aspect of life was neglected, problems surfaced. I have alluded to a few of these problems as David worked with his siblings to decide where Isabel should live and what her care should look like. David's sisters wanted Isabel to remain in her lovely home because they believed she would be happiest at home. Cameron, on the other hand, spoke glowingly of research being done in California in the Bay Area. He thought it might be best to get Isabel out there for more medical tests – where they might even try a new treatment protocol. Cameron and his sisters offered different approaches to certain aspects of their mother's life, but both were missing the complexities of balancing her need for care and quality of life.

All decisions, especially those at the very end of life should be considered life decisions, not simply as one-dimensional medical or physical decisions.

Setting priorities

After a very emotional phone call from one of his siblings, I reminded David that his job as proxy was not to search for consensus each time he approached a decision but to act on his mother's behalf in ways that he believed she would act for herself if she were fully capable of making her own decisions. I asked him point blank, "What do you really want for your mother right now?" I encouraged him to make a list and prioritize it. At this point, Isabel, his beautiful mother, was in a late stage of Alzheimer's. She did not recognize any one, received home care 24/7, ate only what was spooned to her, talked infrequently, and weighed about ninety-five pounds.

An hour or so later, David, came to me with a very short list. Fortunately, he believed that his mother was not suffering or in pain, and she had a medical directive that specified no tube feedings and no use of ventilators at any time. His priorities included safety; good physical care, including hygiene; compassion; and comfort. He ended the list with care that was financially responsible. After five years of 24/7 home care, David and his brother had witnessed a million dollar trust fund dedicated solely to their mother's care dwindle to nothing, and the bank had just informed David that her expense fund was also $35,000 in the red. Clearly, the family needed to think seriously about making alternative arrangements for Isabel's care.

The hour David spent determining goals of care for his mother included weighing the risks and benefits in the four areas that Dr. Ferrell proposes in her quality of life model, namely, the physical, psychological, social, and spiritual dimensions of life. In making his list, David thought through each of these areas, asking all the right questions, and was finally able to begin making the decisions that would insure that her goals of care could be realized.

One thing that David and I learned about home care was that even though home aides were attentive and loyal, they are not always competent regarding the care of persons with Alzheimer's disease. During the five years that Isabel lived at home, we received many calls ranging from stories about Isabel's inappropriate ranting to complaints that the aides were not allowed to take Isabel's dog outside to relieve himself. Because of her paranoia that he would be lost if allowed outside, she had allowed him to soil most of the beautiful

The hour David spent determining goals of care for his mother included weighing the risks and benefits in the four areas that Dr. Ferrell proposes in her quality of life model, namely, the physical, psychological, social, and spiritual dimensions of life.

rugs in her home and even the sofas. We knew that had she been in control of her thoughts she would not have allowed that to happen. Isabel loved and cherished her beautiful furniture and art, and though it didn't directly affect her care, we grieved for her when some of her expensive items were lost, misplaced, or stolen.

As we looked at David's list of goals of care, we knew that Isabel needed care providers who were very savvy about end-stage dementia and who could keep her safe and clean. Friends and family were becoming a scarce commodity in her hometown, and we were no longer sure that she could receive compassionate care there, no matter how much money she had or how much we prayed for it.

We called Cameron, Isabel's oldest son and co-guardian, and one of my favorite men in the entire world. At first, he was very reluctant to consider placing Isabel in an assisted living environment with supplemental care. He had been busy with his own family and had not been back to Oklahoma to witness his mother's increasing frailty and the deterioration of her home.

David told his brother that he thought an assisted living residence would meet the important goal of having her in an environment in which dementia was well understood, especially if we hired supplemental care to help with good hygiene and day-time safety and to provide extra support for feeding her during mealtimes. All in all, by focusing on Betty Ferrell's quality of life framework and asking the right questions, David had found a new and better way to guide Isabel's care in her final days. And Cameron readily agreed to the move when David presented it as the best practical way to focus on what their goals for their mother truly were.

On a cold and icy weekend in December 2007, David, our son Cameron, his girlfriend Beth, and I drove to Bartlesville, Oklahoma. David had gone ahead of us because he wanted to spend time alone with his mother and after doing so, he carried her in her beautiful, full-length fur coat to the car. He had chosen to drive her, himself, to her new home.

Beth, Cameron, and I had spent the morning making her new home look identical to the two rooms in which she had sat and slept in her old house. We furnished it with the same chest, bed and bed linens, and even hung identical art on the walls. It was sad but also rewarding. Her new room was also close to the nursing station so that she would be well attended in the evenings when her supplemental care aides retired for the day.

David told his brother that he thought an assisted living residence would meet the important goal of having her in an environment in which dementia was well understood.

When David carried Isabel's tiny little body into her new and final home, we all felt better. She would be safe, receive impeccable hygienic care on a daily basis, and be assisted at mealtimes. And, eventually, when it was time, hospice would be there to provide the additional comfort and compassion that her sons and daughters desired for her even if they could not be there themselves. When these arrangements had been made, we knew that we had taken the first steps toward accomplishing the newly agreed upon goals of care.

Expect push back

There were bumps in the road, however. We faced one such hurdle a few months later, when David asked his brother to agree to a hospice consultation. We believed that comfort care would be an important end-of-life goal for a person with Isabel's diagnosis and medical directive. But Cameron considered hospice care a last resort and possibly an inappropriate alternative. For him, there was a stigma associated with hospice. It was for cancer patients. Lying in a bed on morphine was not what he desired for his mother. David explained the hospice philosophy to Cameron and described how it could enhance Isabel's care. They agreed to give it a go. She was approaching the final stages of Alzheimer's and easily met hospice criteria.

Not only family members, but also healthcare providers will sometimes push back on the decisions you make for a loved one. After David and his brother agreed to move Isabel and to use goals of care as a way to measure treatment choices, they thoroughly evaluated her medication list and decided that she didn't need to be receiving two anti-dementia drugs. In fact, they decided, she didn't need any anti-dementia drugs. Such drugs are often useful in the early stages of Alzheimer's/dementia, but Isabel had been taking them for over five years, and they were no longer helpful. Many of these medications have gastrointestinal side effects, such as diarrhea; yet Isabel's psychiatrist resisted their decision and actually asked them to put their request to withhold these medications in writing.

David and his brother had moments when they doubted the wisdom of their decision because of the psychiatrist's attitude and her insistence on a written request. Their experience shows that even if you are an experienced healthcare provider and clear about your goals of care, you may have to face down doubts – especially if your decision is to forego an available medical treatment. At such times, Dr. Ferrell's model can be especially helpful.

There were other decisions that David and Cameron made that reflect some of the difficulties encountered when medical treatments do not fit with goals of care. At one point, before Isabel moved to assisted living, her gynecologist discovered that she had an elevated CA-125, a marker for ovarian cancer. David and the gynecologist discussed this at length and David decided that his mother should not have other diagnostic studies. No sonogram. No CT scan. No surgical exploration. Her severely advanced Alzheimer's disease persuaded him that such tests were inappropriate.

David and his brother had moments when they doubted the wisdom of their decision. Their experience shows that even if you are an experienced healthcare provider and clear about your goals of care, you may have to face down doubts – especially if your decision is to forego an available medical treatment.

My sisters and I experienced similar insecurities when we signed a Do-Not-Hospitalize order for our mother three years before she died. After Mother fell several times, we decided that frequent trips to the nearby hospital emergency room were not only unnecessary but also harmful. Were we going to have a CT scan done every time she bumped her head? And if we did opt for a CT scan and it showed something, would we choose neurosurgery for our ninety-year-old mother? We finally agreed that loading Mom into an ambulance and forcing her to wait for hours on a gurney or in a wheelchair in an emergency room was unnecessary. We believed she should be hospitalized only if proper pain control could not be accomplished in the nursing home.

The state of Kansas, where our mother lived, offers this choice, yet our decision was initially resisted by the director of nursing. We reached agreement only after speaking to the social worker and presenting the Kansas "Do Not Hospitalize" form, signed by David, mother's health-care proxy. Choosing not to use a medical modality

Never, ever, did we wish Mom anything but compassion, good care, and safety. Frequent trips to the emergency room were not in keeping with those values.

that is common place can be awkward, even when you know in your heart it is the right thing to do. Never, ever, did we wish Mom anything but compassion, good care, and safety. Frequent trips to the emergency room were not in keeping with those values.

The education of Aunt Mary's proxy

Consider, also, the story of one of my oldest and closest friends Kandy and her seventy-two-year-old Aunt Mary. Aunt Mary had never married and was actually Kandy's father's only sister. Kandy's dad had died at a very young age when Kandy and her sisters were still in high school. Years later, Kandy received a call from a hospital that Aunt Mary had experienced respiratory problems while on her way to play tennis. To save her life, the hospital had intubated Aunt Mary for breathing support. Kandy was informed that she was the designated durable power-of-attorney. Kandy had had little contact with Mary over the last decade and had not known that she was Mary's durable power of attorney for healthcare *and* financial matters. So began Kandy's saga of more than a year of decision making for her aunt.

Upon Mary's arrival at the hospital, she was diagnosed as having pneumonia in addition to chronic asthma. She had suffered with asthma her entire life, so her lungs were damaged and scarred. The emergency room staff had initially tried giving her only oxygen, but soon decided to insert a tube in her throat and place her on a breathing machine or ventilator. She was heavily sedated to help her tolerate the breathing machine and had been admitted to the intensive care unit even before Kandy was notified.

Kandy called me in panic to say the least. How could she make decisions for a woman she hadn't seen in years? "I don't know her," she said. "She's a weird old lady. What am I supposed to do?" After getting the details of the medical situation, I gave her a pep talk. I told her she was in an honorable position. "But get ready for a roller coaster ride," I added.

I knew Kandy well. In her early twenties, Kandy had been diagnosed with malignant melanoma. Her career as a ballerina changed when surgery to treat her cancer entailed stripping her left leg of its lymph nodes. She fought the cancer, however, and later became a dental hygienist. Later, she completed all of her premed requirements but opted for the role of mother instead of doctor. Aunt Mary was no dummy when she chose Kandy to be her healthcare decision maker.

The first thing you have to do, I told her, is build a relationship with the attending doctor and hospitalist. Let him or her know that you will do this job to the best of your ability. Kandy was my roommate in college. I've known her longer than I have known my husband. We are like sisters. She is a brilliant woman but can be very passive. Getting reacquainted with Aunt Mary and navigating the healthcare system would be a new role for this gentle woman.

Then, I told her, you will want to anticipate how one decision leads to another. "Try and think one step ahead," I told her. "Use an 'if' we do this, 'then what' approach to decisions." This kind of procedural approach, I told her, is useful for anticipating the effect that consenting to a treatment or withholding a treatment may have on your aunt's condition. In fact, I encourage everyone to use this approach when communicating with their healthcare team. But for Kandy and Aunt Mary, the slippery slope had begun in the emergency room with the ventilator.

> *The first thing you have to do, I told her, is build a relationship with the attending doctor and hospitalist. Let him or her know that you will do this job to the best of your ability.*

Ten days later, Kandy called me. "Aunt Mary is out of it. It's the only way she can tolerate the ventilator. She can't eat. It's been over a week. I am so confused. The doctor asked me to sign a Do Not Resuscitate (DNR) order but wants to do a tracheotomy. Is that weird?"

I explained why DNR orders are obtained in situations like Mary's. DNR orders are used when a person has an illness of such severity that resuscitation would not be a benefit. I told her that patients in Mary's condition who then suffer an acute heart failure and cannot be brought back to the same level of health that they had before the heart failure would be in an even worse condition if they were resuscitated. Kandy signed the DNR.

"What next?" Kandy asked me. In the case of the tracheotomy, "if" she decided that it was a necessary step, "then" what next? I told her that once her aunt's need for short-term oxygen was addressed, she would have to make decisions about her aunt's short-term nutrition. Mary was receiving feeding through a tube in her nose.

Attempts to wean Aunt Mary from the ventilator failed. The next hurdle was long-term oxygenation and nutrition. Kandy was encouraged to allow a feeding tube to be surgically placed. Weeks went by, and Kandy continued to call me. I frequently asked about Mary's ability to communicate. Even with the use of a pen and paper, Kandy felt Mary was out of touch with the gravity of the situation. Kandy also felt that the hospitalist was not honest with Aunt Mary. When pressed about Mary's prognosis, he would say things like, "My crystal ball is broken." He even told Kandy that he didn't believe Mary could handle the truth. "I don't want to crush her hope at this time," he said. I recommended that Kandy continue to press the doctor to discuss appropriate goals for her aunt, but he would only say, time after time, that her badly damaged lungs merely needed a rest.

As the days crawled by, Kandy lived in constant fear about Mary's future. She had a PEG tube for nutrition, and she was, finally, weaned off the ventilator, but she still required a high level of forced oxygen that could not be delivered in a home setting. She was transferred to a skilled nursing center.

Mary eventually learned to swallow again but remained unable to take adequate nutrition. The feeding tube was never removed. Kandy came to call it the "just-in-case tube," the backup plan. Then, because she was on strong antibiotics, Mary contracted an intestinal bug and suffered from chronic bouts of diarrhea. Her capacity came and went. But fighting for air was such a task that Mary abdicated all decisions to Kandy.

Meanwhile, Kandy discovered her aunt's horrendous financial situation. She appeared to her friends to be living well, but she had incurred tremendous credit card debt. Kandy sent minimal amounts each month to multiple credit card companies. In the end, however, she quit paying Mary's bills. Ruining her credit became the least of Kandy's concerns. Every dime Mary had was needed for her care.

Mary continued to require high levels of forced oxygen but she did learn to walk again. Her mind cleared, friends came to visit, and Kandy tried to talk to Mary about her future. Mary had lived in a one bedroom, upstairs apartment. Her walker and oxygen system would not work there. Kandy was torn between her aunt's fighting spirit and knowing that she could never go home. Kandy finally began to share her concerns with her aunt.

Eventually, Mary was well enough to transfer to a residential care facility. She died there in her sleep. Kandy says her heart was big but it finally gave out. She also says that Mary's denial – that is, her failure to realize her situation – was the only way Mary had found to carry on. Mary's closest friend, Patty, was certain that Mary would get out of the nursing home and move into assisted living. Kandy thought Patty gave Mary false hope, but she also realized that it was a sacred part of their relationship and she did not interfere.

> *Kandy was torn between her aunt's fighting spirit and knowing that she could never go home. Kandy finally began to share her concerns with her aunt.*

I asked Kandy to share with me the lessons she had learned over these eleven months. She was very thoughtful as she described how she learned to give up the micro-managing style she had adopted in the beginning, especially regarding Aunt Mary's money situation. Paying bills on time and preserving her credit appeared initially to be the right thing to do. But very quickly Kandy learned to use Mary's entire retirement income to insure good care.

Kandy also learned a second lesson, namely, how hard it is to predict the future. She still feels ambivalent about how much truth to give a seriously ill and aging person, especially one who is all alone. Kandy's approach to her own cancer years before had been different. She had researched every nook and cranny to learn about her cancer and had even flown to Australia for a surgery that was not certified in the United States. But Aunt Mary was different. She was older, suffering, and needed moral support. "In the end," Kandy said, "not breaking her spirit was as important as maintaining an adequate oxygen level."

> *Aunt Mary was different. She was older, suffering, and needed moral support. "In the end," Kandy said, "not breaking her spirit was as important as maintaining an adequate oxygen level."*

The initial estrangement and distance between these two very different women dissipated over time, and they became close. In the past, Kandy and her family had been critical of Aunt Mary and made negative comments. "She is such a dork. She is so different. Why had she never married? She should have had a family." The final lesson Kandy learned was that Aunt Mary did have a family – and a daughter named Kandy. In the end, Kandy says, "I'm not sure that Aunt Mary fully understood my interpretation of her goals of care. But when she died, she knew that she was loved by me and her closest friends.

Goals of care include more than medical treatment

Kandy's story is unique, but there are many kinds of resistance that healthcare proxies and family may encounter when old friends and acquaintances do not agree with the goals of care that guide their decisions. I often think of my friend and mentor Myra Christopher's experience in caring for her mother-in-law. As the president and CEO of a bioethics center, Myra has dedicated nearly three decades to improving care for the seriously ill and dying. But when her mother-in-law, Mary Frances, was dying, Myra and her husband Truman faced many of the same decisions and obstacles that we all face.

Truman is an only child and was highly involved in his mother's care, even though she lived on her farm in Texas and Myra and Truman lived in Kansas City. When his mother began having frequent falls, Truman felt the usual insecurities about her safety. Mary Frances, however, was a tough, determined Texan. She had been a woman of great independence and had specifically told Myra and Truman not to hospitalize her in her final days. Instead, Truman and Myra requested hospice care for her as her death became imminent.

Several "church women" who were among her friends and visitors did not understand her desire to die at home. They made frequent visits and always commented on her need to go to the hospital. Myra felt such overt resistance and lack of regard for Mary Frances's wishes that she and Truman finally asked the minister to intervene. One of the most vocal of these women was Mary Frances's Sunday-school teacher. The minister, although young and new to town, called the family and assured them that Betty would not be visiting again. He had explained the situation to her and asked her to pray for Mary Frances at home.

For many years, I believed that goals of care were simply medical treatment goals. Then I realized that this equation was missing something, namely, the patient's own voice – the right to choose his or her own medical and life path.

I believe these examples illustrate how useful it is to consider Betty Ferrell's quality of life model as a pattern for making decisions about death and dying. As your parent's health waxes and wanes because of illness and aging, you need to know that the decisions you will make are not only medical decisions. They are also life decisions.

That is why I placed so much emphasis on the importance of knowing your parents' values before you become their proxy or general caregiver or advocate. These values would be the primary decision-making guide if your mom or dad or aunt could speak for him or herself. Many times my mother reminded members of our family and her healthcare team that she wanted to be in an assisted living or nursing home because she valued independence. For her, being independent was a necessary component of the psychological, sociological, and spiritual dimensions of wellness. Even when she was recovering from a bleeding ulcer and was told she couldn't return to assisted living, we knew with confidence that a rehab center was more fitting for her than insisting she spend time recuperating in one of our homes. Even though her health condition and diagnosis precipitated this decision, it was more than a decision to support her physical wellness. It was also the best way to support her need for autonomy.

As your parent's health waxes and wanes because of illness and aging, you need to know that the decisions you will make are not only medical decisions. They are also life decisions.

For many years, I believed that goals of care were simply medical treatment goals. As a young nurse I was taught to begin with subjective data (intuitions) and factor in the objective data (the person's blood pressure, temperature, lab and X-ray results) to arrive at a treatment plan. I was satisfied with that system for the first part of my career, but then I realized that this equation was missing something, namely, the patient's own voice – the right to choose his or her own medical and life path.

The tipping point for me involved the transfer of a ninety-one-year-old man from a nursing home to the hospital where I worked. Three years earlier, he had suffered a stroke that left him unable to speak or walk, and he had lived in the nursing home since that time. Now he had suffered another stroke that caused him to have serious breathing difficulties.

Someone needed to consider the quality of life that Mr. Smith had and to which he would return. What was his long-term prognosis, and what was valuable to him? What benefits would he gain from treatment and what risks would he sustain?

He was given emergency care at the hospital, and subsequently transferred to the intensive care unit (ICU), where I was assigned to be his nurse. I entered the room and found a thin, frail, elderly man with a breathing tube in place that was hooked up to a breathing machine or ventilator. I noted several deep ulcers on his thin hips. As I began to check his pupils as part of my neurological assessment I noticed he had beautiful blue eyes. They reminded me of my father's eyes. As I reviewed the transfer orders from the emergency room, there was a note to set up a central line, a type of IV that enters a large vein in the chest area that can be used for long-term access to a patient for fluids, medications, and nutrition.

As I walked back to the cart to get the central line sterile pack, I felt that this order wasn't a well-thought out procedure. I thought about his blue eyes and how he looked so much like my dad. I looked up the number of the nursing home and called the director. She told me that he was considered an "unbefriended" resident. He had no visitors and had spent much of the last three years in a bed, unable to talk or walk. When propped in a chair, he slumped over. He ate only baby food that was spooned to him. As I hung up the phone, I commented that someone needed to consider the quality of life that Mr. Smith had and to which he would return. What was his long-term prognosis, and what was valuable to him? What benefits would he gain from treatment and what risks would he sustain?

Goals of care represent your loved ones' best interests

The serious nature of these decisions and possible push back from healthcare providers becomes more pressing as the patient approaches the end of life. We understand, of course, that healthcare providers are primarily trained to sustain life. The medical world is all about health, prevention, and cure; I have no complaints about that. But there comes a time when family and healthcare providers must make an honest appraisal of what goals of care are in the best interests of the dying patient. Then your parent's wishes and values are important – indeed, they trump – all other considerations.

There comes a time when family and healthcare providers must make an honest appraisal of what goals of care are in the best interests of the dying patient.

Exploring your parents' goals of care is the most important thing that you can do for them. It is certainly the most valuable lesson that David and I learned, and it was then that I began to live up to the name a director of nursing had given me nearly two decades earlier. She had called me a "charming troublemaker." As I prodded David, my own sisters, and all those working in long-term care facilities to question their usual ways of thinking and doing things, I lovingly shook their worlds. I hope after reading this chapter, that you will have the courage and patience to do that for your parents.

Weighing the risks and benefits of where your loved ones will live, who will care for them, what medicines they will take, and what medical interventions are right for them will no doubt require you to swim upstream. You will be the one asking difficult questions and challenging the benefits to be gained from the usual or standard treatment. You will need to become a "charming troublemaker" in your family and healthcare systems, and, at times, among your parents' circle of friends and community. The task of marrying the wonders of modern medicine to the values and healthcare wishes of your family members in their quest for quality of life and a good death is a task worthy of your finest effort.

> *The task of marrying the wonders of modern medicine to the values and healthcare wishes of your family members in their quest for quality of life and a good death is a task worthy of your finest effort.*

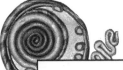

Lessons for Living without Regrets

- As a proxy or family decision maker, you will be asked to help determine goals of care for your loved ones.

- Consider your parents' values and wishes and what you hope to accomplish on their behalf.

- Use goals of care to determine what you *should* do, not what you *can* do.

- A rule of thumb for setting goals of care: Think it through. "If we do this now, what is next?"

- End-of-life decisions are really life decisions and include not only the physical aspects of well-being, but also the social, spiritual, and psychological dimensions of well-being.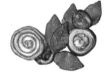

- Repeat goals of care planning intermittently with each change in your parents' health status.

CHAPTER 7

Caregiving
Many Roles, Many Star Players

When I was in the sixth grade, my classroom teacher asked her students to write biographical reports on someone we considered a hero. Most of my friends reported on their favorite U.S. president or sports legend. Not I. I wrote about Clara Barton, the famous Civil War nurse and legendary founder of the American Red Cross. Even at an early age, I was enamored with caregivers and considered caregiving to be one of my strengths or gifts. I have always loved people, and I like helping them feel better, whether they are ill or not.

Why then did I find myself struggling to write this chapter on caregiving? After several days of muddling around in my head, I finally realized that I was still struggling with not having provided direct care to my mother when she was no longer able to live in her own home. Instead, she chose to live with my younger sister's family about five miles from my home. And David was not a "hands-on" caregiver for his mother or for Karen, his disabled sister. Both Karen and his mother were cared for by paid caregivers. How important, then, can our advice be on this very important topic? Were we really caregivers even though we did not bathe, feed, or administer daily care to our mothers?

My inner turmoil caused me to think more honestly about what really defines a caregiver. It also helped me to articulate what

I really wanted to accomplish in this chapter. I resolved to do more than teach the facts about families in America who provide care to their family members. My goals in this chapter are to help you understand a variety of caregiver roles and to envision the impact that caregiving will have on you and your family. I want you to know that even if you are primarily involved in the decision making aspect of care – as David and I were – you may also be called on to offer "hands on" assistance. Being ready for that call can greatly enhance the experience.

Even if you are primarily involved in the decision making aspect of care – as David and I were – you may also be called on to offer "hands on" assistance. Being ready for that call can greatly enhance the experience.

An elusive and multifaceted reality

On any given day in the United States, one in four people – about 65.7 million individuals – provide informal care on a full or part-time basis to either a spouse or a parent. Further, as described by the National Alliance for Caregiving (2009), many of these caregivers are females about 48 years old who work full-time and yet spend a minimum of twenty hours in the caregiver role. If these numbers seem unbelievable, think about how many of your friends and family members already fill these shoes, and as our population ages, these numbers are likely to increase. Do you see caregiving in your future?

The definitions of caregiver are nearly as staggering as the data are elusive and multilayered. Official descriptions range from acute or episodic caregivers who generally tend to others only in a crisis to chronic caregivers who provide ongoing care during lengthy illnesses or disabilities. The care we give to aging parents usually begins as episodic and progresses to ongoing care over time.

Caregiving may also be described as formal or informal. Formal caregiving includes compensation or payment; informal caregiving is provided by friends and family who are not formally paid. Though these distinctions may seem trivial, it is important to realize that somewhere, sometime, someone in your family will need your help whether you are a trained healthcare provider or not, and the odds are that you will not be compensated. All of us are or will eventually be called on to do things for others that they cannot do for themselves, but nowhere is the role of caregiving more overwhelming than when we are caring for an aging parent.

As the roles of family caregivers expand, so do the time commitments. Bell curves are used on many websites to make this point.

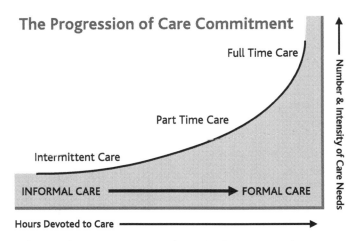

Adapted from www.heartwarmingcare.com/understanding-the-progression-of-care-commitment.
Posted by Randy Walden, September 1, 2008.

Caregiving usually begins with a few phone calls and infrequent errands, then ramps up to more frequent requests for help, including, for example, transportation to doctor appointments, grocery shopping, meal preparation, and picking up and managing medications. As time progresses, you may need to plan more frequent visits to your parents' home (whether next door, across town, across the state, or across the country). You will need to see them to assess changes in their mental and physical status. As the need for care escalates, you may receive calls in the night alerting you that your loved one has fallen or is in distress. He or she may need emergency care or hospitalization. If you are working, you may need family leave time so that you can stay with them when they return home after such episodes. As their health issues compound, you may ask them to move closer to you to make care more readily accessible. You get the picture. The caregiver's role constantly increases in complexity and challenge.

Caregiving usually begins with a few phone calls and infrequent errands, then ramps up to more frequent requests for help.

In retrospect, David and I began as informal caregivers to our mothers when we were in our early forties. His mother lived about three hours from our Kansas City home. My mother resided in Kansas City. More than a decade of informal caregiving ensued as both Mable's and Isabel's physical and mental health changed. What began as an honor – that is, as something we felt good about – gradually became more burdensome. We were often bone weary and frustrated by how much they seemed to expect from us.

In the beginning, we said to each other and to friends that "we wouldn't have it any other way." We felt a sense of pride that we were caring for the women who had meant the most to us. But as years rolled by, we whispered under our breath, "What are we doing? When will this end? Where are the troops?" In no way had we understood what we were getting into. We lost weight, battled insomnia, and fought with other family members and each other.

Only when I read Lee Woodruff's book, *In an Instant*, did I realize how universal our experience was. Indeed, very few families escape this world without suffering one or several unexpected health crises that may require as much family healing as physical treatment and healing for the member who is injured, ill, or dying. Lee Woodruff captures the intensity of this effect. She writes that the explosion that nearly killed her husband was not only an unanticipated health crisis for him but an event that threatened to blow their entire family apart.

You may recall that Bob Woodruff, an immensely popular journalist for the ABC television network, was seriously injured in Iraq in 2006. He was hit by an improvised explosive device (IED) and suffered serious and extensive brain trauma. The injury was so severe that he was induced into a coma and his survival listed as doubtful. Lee, a young wife and mother, precipitously and instantly became the healthcare proxy for her husband and a single parent. Her real work, as she describes it in this family memoir, was

In the beginning, we said to each other and to friends that "we wouldn't have it any other way." But as years rolled by, we whispered under our breath, "What are we doing? When will this end? Where are the troops?"

to put back together what the IED had blown apart: her husband, his future, and their entire family. She used the physical metaphor of what Bob lived through to describe what happened, simultaneously, to her life and family. The byline of her memoir is captioned, "A Family's Journey of Love and Healing." Bob and the entire Woodruff family needed a year of rehabilitation before Bob could return to journalism and his family to life.

As I read her story, I felt a deep emotional pull. I thought "she's got it right!" Not that aging, even with its inevitable declines, bears any resemblance to the trauma of an unexpected explosion. Far from it: aging is a normal part of life, and its last quarter is a time to savor our accomplishments, our relationships, and the wisdom that we may have accrued. Nevertheless, our mortality remains; our energy and physical strength decrease and our dependence on family and friends increases. Often, the changes are subtle, until suddenly, perhaps after a fall or a stroke or trouble with breathing, the problem erupts and the entire family is thrown into a tailspin. Then healing must occur, not only for our parents' but also for the family members who care for them.

> *Aging is a normal part of life, and its last quarter is a time to savor. Nevertheless, our mortality remains; our energy and physical strength decrease and our dependence on family and friends increases.*

Caregivers are on their own perilous journey with all its hidden trials and tribulations. They, too, are ill at times and yearn for wellness. Caregiving is what we *do* for our mothers or fathers or other loved ones, but it is also a striving for balance and resiliency. To do it well, we must (1) learn to take care of ourselves (individually), and (2) strive (together) to reach a new equilibrium and stability in the family. David and I had a lot of that to do in our effort to be authentic and compassionate caregivers.

Caregiving's emotional and physical tolls

In the decade of our mothers' declines, our eldest child, Cameron, then in his twenties, was diagnosed with a very serious illness. He was in Kansas City hospitals more than a dozen times over a two-year period and at Mayo Clinic for two major surgeries. Looking back, I realize that David and I had never in our healthcare careers experienced so much stress and lack of preparation as we did in becoming family caregivers.

Soon after his college graduation, Cameron was suddenly, inexplicably, disabled by an autoimmune, intestinal disease. Until then, he had been the very picture of good health, always the captain of his high school football and basketball teams. For some time, his condition was undiagnosed. His weight dropped to less than 150 pounds, down at least twenty-five pounds from healthier times. His red blood counts were dangerously low, and at one point, he experienced as many as thirty bloody stools per day. Doctors finally diagnosed his illness as ulcerative colitis.

For weeks at a time, David and I moved out of the master suite in our home and slept on a nearby pull-out sofa while Cameron lay in our big bed receiving intravenous nutrition. At one time, he was not allowed to eat for thirty days. David continued to work long, hard hours. I cared for Cameron. His sisters, Maggie and Libby were away at Northwestern and Skidmore Colleges. The telephone rang incessantly; calls came in about David's mother and mine. On good days we joked that our version of being part of the sandwich generation looked more like a super-sized hoagie – too big to chew unless taken in small bites.

David and I had never in our healthcare careers experienced so much stress and lack of preparation as we did in becoming family caregivers.

All we could do was put one foot in front of the other each day. We didn't think about the journey, we just plodded along. Only later, when Cameron's health improved, would we say we had *trudged*. The many tasks involved in family caregiving became our daily lives and could not be reassigned to others.

During this time, many of our closest friends were also providing support to their aging parents. We tried to listen and offer our best advice and support. For example, Mary, one of my dearest friends, often talked to David and me about her dad. He had – has – Parkinson's syndrome, and the drugs for Parkinson's cause Pat all kinds of other problems: incontinence, constipation, and a debilitating weakness. Before retiring and before Parkinsonism, this father of eight had been a successful commodities broker. He was and is an Irish Catholic, full of fun and jolly – the kind of man his son-in-law, Morgan, calls, an Irish leprechaun. He is generous to everyone around him. But after retiring and battling Parkinson's disease, Pat became impossible to please and was especially intractable for Cathy, his late wife, though she cared for him with tenderness and patience.

On several occasions, David and I traveled with Mary and her husband to visit her sister Carol in Florida. Pat and Cathy often joined us on these visits. We younger couples played golf, cooked out, or dined at a great seafood restaurant, always enjoying the mild weather and good conversation. But it was difficult to ignore how much attention and maintenance their dad required. He didn't feel well. His computer wouldn't work. He needed a ride some place. Where were his golf shorts?

His wife looked downtrodden and, many times, depressed. She often sat on the back porch, watching an outdoor television, completing crossword puzzles, and smoking. Her daughters would become exasperated – with Cathy as much as with their dad.

Since I love to sneak a cigarette every now and again, I had a perfect opportunity to talk with Cathy. She was a strong-willed Italian woman married to an irascible Irish Catholic. She and Pat had shared many highs in their married life (great kids, wealth, good friends, beautiful homes), and some low points (Pat had been an alcoholic for years before getting sober, and some of their grown children had divorced). During our time on the porch, I learned that

Pat had always been in the spotlight for one reason or another, and it looked to me like he intended to stay right there even as he aged.

After the six of us golfed, we returned home long enough to shower and choose the evening restaurant. Cathy stayed behind to enjoy her favorite glass of white wine and eat leftovers, even if Pat joined us for a dinner outing. Over the last few years, she lost weight. She coughed. She said she was fine. But eventually, she was diagnosed with lung cancer. She lived only two weeks after she was officially diagnosed. For reasons no one will ever understand, she chose to forgo an earlier diagnosis. She denied her own needs as she and the family worked tirelessly to manage Pat's care.

In the end, she called each of her grown children to her bedside and spoke with them individually. She tidied up the past and shared her hopes for their future. Her words were honest, comforting, and clarifying. She was the ultimate

> *In the end, she called each of her grown children to her bedside and spoke with them individually. She tidied up the past and shared her hopes for their future.*

caregiver. She had raised eight children, including five, wild, Irish sons. And she cared for her husband. To have done otherwise would have been unthinkable to a woman like Cathy Hennessy.

Pat now has round-the-clock care in his private home in Chicago, where seven of his children still live. His daughter Carol is his healthcare proxy, but I believe it takes all hands on deck to handle Pat! The Hennessy family, like most families, struggle with the daily details of managing his care. And, sadly, it has taken a toll on their family, especially since Cathy's death. They do their trudging, as David and I did, with heavy hearts but heads held high. Their work as family caregivers is not finished. One of

Cathy's best legacies is the love and strength her children give their dad when it is needed.

The importance of self-care

David and I were somewhat crippled after Cameron's illness and our mothers' deaths. We sold our big house and moved into a beautiful condominium, only to flail in our marriage. We talked to a counselor who was surprised that after all we'd been through; the worst thing we could tell him about our marriage is that we were unkind to one another. Did we have affairs? Did we abuse alcohol or drugs? Did we lie to one another? We sat there in his office, laughing through our tears and shook our heads. "Who has time to have an affair or think up meanness?"

During ten years of caring for our mothers, extended families, and children, we had forgotten how to take emotional and physical care of ourselves. My blood pressure was high and David had to struggle to save enough time just to get his hair cut or his teeth cleaned. It took a year of counseling before we realized how long it had been since we didn't feel like we were "on call" for our aging mothers or Cameron. (Of course, much of that time David really was on call.)

During ten years of caring for our mothers, extended families, and children, we had forgotten how to take emotional and physical care of ourselves.

Recently at a Sunday church service, David and I observed a new cohort of chaplains taking oaths for the upcoming year. Most of the creed they recited sounded reasonable and centered on the things they would do as pastoral, prayerful, intercessors. But one thing they pledged really surprised me. They promised, publicly, before a church audience, to "practice self-care." I looked at David and whispered, "How unusual." But as I sat there, I thought about caregiving, about chaplaincy, and then about our lives. How helpful would it have been had we made that same promise to one another as we cared for our family, friends, and one another? The chaplains' oath and Lee Woodruff's book serve as enlightening moments about our experience as caregivers. Both contain a lesson important enough to be passed on to you and others – namely, the importance of taking care of oneself while caring for others.

Learning how to be a caregiver

My friend and colleague Sandy is an elder care attorney who has administered many professional caregiving initiatives in Kansas City. Over dinner, recently, I asked her to tell me what caregivers really need to know. I told her that I wanted to share the "best of the best" with the readers of this book. Her years of experience in the field reveal that there are three critical aspects of caregiving.

First, she advises us to identify ourselves as caregivers as early in the process as possible. It is empowering to recognize at the very start of the journey that caregiving behavior is a social phenomenon though its manifestations are unique to each individual and its complexities manifold. Second, be aware that caregiving is skill-based behavior and that exercising these skills may have little to do with other skills that you developed in your relationships – for example, as mother, daughter, niece, aunt, or uncle. Indeed, many of your earlier skills may be turned on end when caregiving becomes the focus. The third important aspect of caregiving, according to Sandy, is the building of a supportive network, but this task is only possible after you have successfully negotiated the first two steps.

Many siblings and spouses do not think about caregiving until they find themselves in the hall of the hospital trying to figure out what to do now that the discharge plan requires that someone – and who, if not you? – must accept this role before your loved one can to be allowed to return home. Everyone in the family system may have known that Mom or Dad or Uncle Bob was one incident or serious illness away from needing care. But it is easy to deny or ignore an acute episode until a hospitalization threatens to change their lives or yours. David and I seemed to have skipped this step. There was no official moment that defined us as caregivers. We were years into that role with our mothers before the implications became clear. In fact, as I confessed earlier, with my mother, though not with our son, I was unsure about what my role in her care should be.

Many siblings and spouses do not think about caregiving until they find themselves in the hall of the hospital trying to figure out what to do now...

Maybe David and I were naive, thinking that because we were from big families, we would not be called to be caregivers. Surely our older siblings would claim that role. Or maybe we thought that nurturing a young family and building our careers were our primary roles and responsibility. We only saw what was right in front of us.

Sandy shared her own story with me about becoming a caregiver for her father. Ben was in relatively good health when his wife died. He was a go-getter and "nothing ventured, nothing gained" was his personal motto. But growing up in the coal mines of Pennsylvania and smoking during much of his adult life took a toll on his health. Living independently in Dearborn, Michigan, became challenging after lung surgery, prostate complications, and, finally, lung malignancy.

Sandy, a dedicated daughter and expert in the field of elder law and caregiving, stepped outside both roles when she said to Ben on the phone, "Please move to Kansas City. I want you to be close by when you need more than I can offer you long-distance." Luckily for Sandy, Ben did just that. He made a new life here. He bowled. He cut his grass and hers.

Ben agreed that Sandy should attend his medical appointments, but that was not when she officially became his caregiver. Even when his vision deteriorated and he began experiencing shortness of breath, he remained quite independent. Sandy did insist that he not climb the ladder to trim the trees unless she were there to hold the ladder, but all in all, their relationship was that of father and daughter.

Ben had a unique system for mowing his lawn. He placed a lawn chair in a particular spot on the driveway from which he could mow a few rows at a time and rest in between. Eventually, the mowing project became a task lasting several days. "Why should I pay someone to do something I can do on my own!" he complained to Sandy. On one particularly hot and humid Kansas City summer day, Sandy sneaked over to Ben's home and mowed his lawn. She realized that day that her dad was laboring against odds that would surely not weigh in his favor at some point. As she mowed the grass, she realized that she was doing something for her Dad that he had always done for himself. She said, "It's better to know now – sooner rather than later – that I am not just Ben's daughter, but also his caregiver."

Ben agreed that Sandy should attend his medical appointments, but that was not when she officially became his caregiver.

Sandy's story demonstrates the differences between being a caregiver and loving someone who needs care. Essentially, she claims that sustaining loving relationships or caring about another does not mean that we are prepared to be caregivers. A caregiver, she says, must gather information and master tasks.

Even though you may be the best daughter in the entire world, you may not be able to perform a myriad of caregiving tasks. For example, your ability to care can be constrained by time demands in your own life. I recall that early on in my mother's care, her driving abilities became an issue as her vision and physical strength declined. At the onset of becoming her driver, my sisters and I shared the responsibilities. We laughed and referred to our turns as "driving Miss Mable." But over time, as Mom became dependent on us for all her transportation – not just for doctor appointments, but for taking her to church and even to visit other siblings and her grandchildren – things became complicated. Being a loving daughter was not the same as being a chauffeur.

As roles escalate, so do skill sets. As our parents age, their health declines and they may have trouble walking, which can affect their ability to bathe safely or to prepare meals. At one point, my sisters and I decided that daily meal delivery was an important intervention if Mom wanted to continue living in her own home.

Medication protocols can also be very challenging – difficult to understand and to deliver properly. Would you be willing not only to count pills but also to deliver injections to an aging parent? Would you be willing to help your parent with toileting and hygiene needs? And even if you are willing to provide this level of care, would your Mom or Dad want you to help them with these tasks? Clearly, some conversation and soul searching may be needed to understand your feeling or change your parents' way of thinking.

At one time, after Mom chose to live with my younger sister Cinda, it became evident that Cinda's own health was preventing her from fulfilling all the responsibilities that caregiving entails. Cinda has often battled depression, which is probably why Mom chose to live with her, at least initially. Mom needed care but she was also still deep into giving care: she wanted to be there for Cinda when Cinda needed her. Over time, questions, even conflicts about meal preparation, soiled bed clothing, and Mom's frequent falls helped us realize that another intervention was necessary. Between her depression and caring for Mom, Cinda was drowning in too many responsibilities. It had nothing to do with not loving Mom enough. Cinda not only had to face the fact that our mother's health was declining, she also had to deal with her own health issues. Her health and Mom's health and safety became our priorities. The multifaceted aspects of caring are emotional as well as physical.

One of the major skills of caregiving is knowing when such transitions are necessary – especially if the transition involves a new housing arrangement (this important topic will be discussed in more detail in our next chapter). We helped Cinda manage this transition by constantly reminding her that loving Mom was separate from caring for her daily needs. We all treasured Cinda's

> *Sandy's story demonstrates the differences between being a caregiver and loving someone who needs care … A caregiver, she says must gather information and master tasks.*

ability to manage Mom's finances and the piles of paperwork that are common in the care of an aging parent, and Cinda never let us down regarding that aspect of Mom's care.

Rallying the troops

Recall my friend Sandy's third critical aspect of caregiving, and shout it from the rooftops: build a supportive network! Sandy reminded me that when a new child is announced, we rally. We take food. We shower the new family with love, gifts, and our time.

Families with a declining member need similar support. They, like mothers of newborns, need help with daily, ordinary tasks – not because an aging member is the same as a newborn, but because the caregiver faces expanding roles and responsibilities, which quite frankly, overtake them much more suddenly than a baby's nursery can be equipped.

I follow a website called "Top Tips to Help Aging Parents" written by Janice Wallace. She calls herself a Caregiving Coach because her mission is to teach viewers how to be successful caregivers. In one of her posts, she reveals that in her caregiving years, she was often defensive if anyone asked her if she needed help. Did they think she wasn't or couldn't handle her responsibilities? Did they think they could do a better job? She says that when you are literally "on a roll" "in your role" you become pretty darn good at what has to be done and others can let you down by not performing in ways that meet your expectations.

Janice believes that caregiving frequently requires asking others for assistance. Friends and family can and will often help, especially if we are very clear and articulate about what we need.

Nevertheless, doing it all has its limitations. In the end, Janice believes that caregiving frequently requires asking others for assistance. Friends and family can and will often help, especially if we are very clear and articulate about what we need from them.

Contributing to the care of an aging parent is multidimensional and many times has that familiar feeling of taking two steps forward and three steps back until we figure out what is really needed. But whether you are a primary caregiver or a loving family member, paying attention to what your aging family member really needs requires a huge sense of dedication. You may need to pitch in to make the aging person's life better or you may be more successful in supporting those who are providing direct care for your loved ones. Learn what it is that you do best, and lean on others for support.

Throughout this book are stories showing how intently and often patients, friends, and family relied on David and me for advice regarding healthcare decisions involving their aging parents. We were part of their troops, yet there were times subsequently that we found ourselves ill prepared for making decisions and caring for our own mothers.

> *Learn what it is that you do best and lean on others for support.*

Looking back, we realize that at different times in our caregiving experience, we, too, had to call in the troops – not only other family members but also individuals that we called our outside experts. When, for example, Isabel began showing signs of memory loss and confusion, we asked a geriatric case manager to help us evaluate her ability to live safely in her own home. This expert made several safety suggestions, including placing guard rails in the bathroom shower and removing throw rugs to prevent falls. Without her help, we would have had no idea how to make a home safe for an aging person.

At times I tease our three children about what their roles will be when they care for me in my aging days. I imagine that Libby, our middle child, will be the one who tries, single-handedly, to care for me in her home, even if she has a house full of children, dogs, cats, a career, and a busy husband. Cameron, our son and a finance guy, will hold everyone's feet to the fire regarding my expenses and remind everyone of what his dad would have said. And, the youngest, Maggie, now in training to be a doctor, will make sure that I am not on too many medications and remind Libby, as I did Cinda, that being a loving daughter is not the same as providing daily care for me.

The rest of my story as an aging woman will be written by the people who love me and will do for me what I will no longer be able to do for myself, just as David and I did for our aging mothers, and at times, our son. The hope I have for my children then will be the same hope I now extend to you. May you discover in these pages a few helpful tools that can make your caring less a drudgery than a long satisfying run for which you are well prepared.

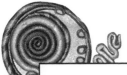

Lessons for Living without Regrets

- The care we give to aging parents usually begins as episodic and progresses to ongoing care over time.

- Caregiving begins when we begin doing things for our mothers or fathers or other loved ones that they can no longer do for themselves.

- Caregivers often have a hard time caring for themselves and remembering that they too are searching for wellness.

- Three important steps in caregiving:
  - Identify and accept yourself as caregiver as early in the process as possible.
  - Understand that being a caregiver is not the same as being a loving son or daughter. Caregivers have different responsibilities and require different skills.
  - Build a supportive network!

CHAPTER 8

Choosing Mom and Dad's Last Home
Compassionate Care and Justice

I have known my friend Judy for twenty-five years and I have never seen her when she didn't look exquisite, whether golfing, out for dinner, or even casually shopping at the grocery store. She was the ladies' golf champion at our country club for more than a dozen years. She never talks about her age, aches, pains, or family issues, though I know she had a brother, Jack, who died tragically in a car wreck hurrying to get his college date home and meet curfew. Her father, Jim Geisendorf, owned a funeral home in Salina, Kansas, where both he and her mother Marjorie were civic leaders beloved by the entire community. Judy and her husband Charlie have always been extremely loyal to her parents. They seemed to be always headed for Salina to play golf or celebrate the holidays. Many times I have forgotten that the Geisendorfs were Judy's adored parents; they were more like best friends.

During the last ten years Jim suffered from macular degeneration and lost much of his vision. He and Marjorie downsized from their large home to a condominium in an adult aging community. Both were becoming less independent as they aged. By the time they were in their ninth decade, Judy and Charlie had assumed many of the informal caregiving roles we discussed in chapter seven.

Last year for the Easter holiday, Charlie and Judy drove to Salina and took her parents out for Mexican fare and margaritas

(Marjorie's favorite cocktail). It was the night before Easter. That night, while sleeping, Jim suffered a massive heart attack and died peacefully in the hospital a few hours later on Easter morning. The months since his death have become increasingly challenging for Charlie and Judy. It is a rare Saturday morning that Marjorie doesn't call Judy for help: "I'm confused." "I don't know what to do today." "I'm just so stupid."

Often when Marjorie calls Judy, she sounds upset and frightened and insists that Judy come as soon as possible – "right now" – but when they arrive, she's dressed for the day, relaxed, and greets them without any signs of distress! Judy and Charlie respond to her with great love and devotion. Nevertheless, the three-hour drive, which so often proves unnecessary, has become cumbersome and wearing.

Marjorie, now ninety-five years old, takes only one medication. She needs a walker and her short-term memory is failing, but she is a healthy aging woman. She had always worked with her husband in the family's business, but when I asked Judy what her mother had done professionally, she couldn't remember what her mother's title had been. Basically, Marjorie was so organized and bright that she hadn't needed a title or a job description. She had always been at the helm of their family. Five years ago, when Judy began planning her mother's ninetieth birthday celebration, she asked Marjorie how many invitations she should order to include Marjorie's closest friends. Marjorie calmly replied that 200 would be about right. Sure enough, when Judy received the mailing list, it contained 199 names. They eventually held two open houses for her birthday celebration.

More recently, Judy and Charlie have begun asking questions about where Marjorie should live. They realize that the days Marjorie had formerly spent caring for her husband are now very empty and lonely. They also wonder if her memory loss is worsening or if Jim had been covering for her as she had compensated for his visual impairment. "How many times can we speed down that highway?" "Should Marjorie live closer to us?" "Does she need assistance?" "What if she falls?" "Is she depressed as well as lonely?"

Judy's questions are the same questions many of us face or will face when one parent dies and the other is left alone. And no question is more difficult for the surviving parent and his or her children to decide. Where will Mom live now that she's alone?

Helping your parents' choose their final home is difficult because it is an emotional question. It may be that no one – not you or your parents – can discuss it dispassionately, and it is not a stand-alone decision. It is closely related to your earlier and larger discussions about your parents' goals of care (see chapter 6). Fortunate, indeed, are the families who face this question early in their conversations, but even so, your parents' need for continuing independence and your concern for their safety and need to preserve your own autonomy make this decision a delicate issue. You may think that serious illness, loss of capacity, and death and dying are the hard issues, but as David and I worked with our mothers and families, it became clear to us that medical and health-related decisions are likely to be less emotionally loaded than decisions regarding our parents' living arrangements.

> *Helping your parents' choose their final home is difficult because it is an emotional question. . . . Fortunate, indeed, are the families who face this question early in their discussions.*

Healthcare treatments are primarily dictated by the patient's illness and its trajectory. For example, when a parent is actively dying, decisions regarding pain management, comfort care, and when to provide supplemental oxygen must be considered. If a parent has end-stage dementia, his or her nutritional needs and safety must also be considered. Even decisions to forgo aggressive care and allow comfort measures to ease your parents' dying can often be rationally discussed. But housing considerations are unlikely to be weighed early in the process.

In this chapter, I will present the questions that David and I and our friends confronted in our quest to make the right housing choices for our aging parents. Our answers may vary, but the questions, we soon discovered, are the same questions that every family asks in this situation: How do these decisions relate to your established goals of care? Who will be included in the conversation as you sift the options? What factors besides health should be considered and – most important – how do we set our priorities? Is there a trump card to help us narrow the options? Is peace of mind attainable?

No Easy Answers

For several semesters I have co-taught a university course on the biological and bioethical issues of aging. The university sits in an urban setting and has a diverse student population. One recent class included several Latin American students and many Asian and southeast Asian students. During a discussion about long-term care and aging in America, many of these students talked about their grandparents or great-grandparents. A vigorous debate ensued as several students voiced their opinion that many families in our country don't take care of their own. One student specifically said that "American families desert and abandon their aging parents and place them in nursing homes only to forget about them and go their merry way."

No doubt students always reflect their own cultural perspectives, and these students believe that compassionate care is best learned from past generations and from watching their own parents care for their grandparents. One Hispanic student told us that his current home held four generations! But other students argued that in their families, the responsibilities of caregiving, including time and the need for specialty medical care, are more than their working parents can safely provide. I was surprised that the conversation of these twenty-year-olds touched on the contentious issues that David and I had faced when we had to decide where our mothers would be most comfortable and best cared for during their last years of life. Though David and I share the same ethnic background, our families of origin have different notions of what is and isn't culturally acceptable.

These classroom discussions were an opportunity for teaching the goals of applied ethics. Each student could see first-hand that different families could reach different results and still be acting ethically. Ethics, I told them, demands respect for values and cultural mores and an acknowledgment that each situation is unique. "There is a difference between agreement and acceptance," I told them. "Accepting what a family is doing for its loved ones does not mean that you agree with

I wanted these students to realize that each situation is unique and that each person must learn to see the other person's side in weighing this difficult issue.

its decisions, but it does mean acknowledging the family's right to engage in a thoughtful process and make the decision that is right for a particular situation." I wanted these students to realize that each situation is unique and that each person must learn to see the other person's side in weighing this difficult issue. Different choices can be made about long-term care and residential placement, especially when cultural differences are acknowledged and respected.

Ethics courses are challenging for many students because ethical dilemmas do not have clear, unambiguous answers. Students and indeed all of us are more comfortable if our thinking yields measurable outcomes such as we encounter in science, math, technology, or economics. But working with family members and healthcare providers to make moral or ethical choices with and for your parents rarely results in a perfect or simple solution. I can think of no magical formula that can help you decide where your mom or dad should live in their final days or where you and your family will say your final goodbyes. But with understanding and active listening, you can find the solution that is best for your family at this time.

Health status, financial resources, and housing options

Although you will not find an easy methodology for choosing the right housing choice for your loved one, a consideration of three factors can help keep your emotions in check. First, consider your parents' or aging loved ones' current health status, including their mental and physical conditions, and involve them in the decision-making process. If they have capacity or intermittent periods of capacity, their voices belong at the heart of the discussion. Sadly, however, fear of some housing options may keep them silent. Be prepared to acknowledge these fears and work through them as various options are presented. In my family, I was the lucky one. My mother's voice guided this decision from the beginning, and she transitioned from her home to my sister's, to assisted living, to the hospital and rehabilitation, to living her final years in a small, privately owned nursing home.

Second, consider your family's financial resources. Does the family have funds that can be applied to their housing needs? Recall that David's mother Isabel had access to private insurance, Medicare, and trust funds. My mother had only Medicare and Medicaid benefits. Although their financial situations represent opposing ends of the financial continuum, resource assessment was an essential consideration for both mothers and should never be ignored.

Third, after examining your parent's health and financial standings, explore the options for housing that exist in your family and in the community. Can they remain in their own home with assistance? Should they live with you in your home or with a sibling? Do they need to live in a skilled nursing facility or in a senior living community? You will want to consider settings ranging from independent living, to assisted living, to skilled nursing as well as with special units for persons with Alzheimer's/dementia and memory loss. Regardless of the setting, size, cost, or location, each of these options has a marketing director ready to offer you a splendid deal.

Consider your parents' or aging loved ones current health status, including their mental and physical conditions, and involve them in the decision-making process. If they have capacity or intermittent periods of capacity, their voices belong at the heart of the discussion.

When you have addressed your parents' preferences, health status, financial capacity, and the community options available to them, you will be ready to consider which of these settings is most likely to give your family maximum comfort and peace of mind. The final measuring stick that David and I used throughout the spectrum of decisions we faced was to search out the choice that would honor our parents' goals and values and cause the least regrets in the long term.

At this time, you may want to read or review your parents' goals of care (see chapter 6). Then you can explore the medical options and protocols that a potential dwelling offers to determine which ones really fit your parents' needs and goals. Most decisions about housing are made when serious decline is occurring or has occurred, but even if your parents are not critically ill, you will need to approach this decision based on their current health concerns and in anticipation of what the next step in their healthcare trajectory is likely to be. Your parents' health may pass through temporary peaks and valleys, but you will be wise to prepare for increasing frailty.

Practical questions about your parents' mobility and their ability to obtain proper nutrition should be considered as well as changes in their capacity and agility. It is also a practical matter to assess their need for supplemental oxygen, daily blood sugar testing, help with organizing and remembering to take their daily medications, toileting assistance, and hygiene. Such considerations will present a fairly accurate picture of how much support your parents need. Alterations in mental status and capacity present immense barriers to Mom's or Dad's ability to live independently. The more they require assistance, the more they will need stronger support than most independent living facilities can offer.

The final measuring stick that David and I used throughout the spectrum of decisions we faced was to search out the choice that would honor our parents' goals and values and cause the least regrets in the long term.

Acute illnesses or a new, more serious diagnosis can serve as a tipping point triggering a housing decision or change in residence. Recall my friend Kandy's experience in caring for her Aunt Mary. Kandy only learned that she was her Aunt Mary's healthcare proxy when her aunt suffered an acute case of pneumonia, but this episodic pneumonia led to more than a year of ebbs and flows in Mary's health status. Kandy soon faced a wide array of decisions – life and death decisions regarding breathing machines for her aunt, decisions regarding her need for long-term, high levels of oxygen, and decisions about artificial nutrition on both a temporary and long-term basis.

As Mary's health continued to decline, she resided in three different facilities, although Kandy continued to maintain her small apartment. Initially Mary was in the intensive care unit of the hospital. Later she was moved to the step-down unit from intensive care, then to a medical-surgical floor within the hospital. Finally, Mary was discharged from the hospital, but because she was dependent on a feeding tube and ventilator, Kandy found her a place in a facility that supported intense medical needs. As time passed, however, and Aunt Mary recuperated ever so slightly, Kandy returned to the drawing board and found her a less restrictive residential care facility. My point in reviewing Kandy's story with you is that the medical needs your parents have are an important consideration and often begin a domino-like cascade of decisions culminating in having to choose where your loved one will reside.

Novel solutions are possible

Kandy's family currently offers another helpful story regarding housing choices. Guy Furman, Kandy's step-dad, became severely ill the weekend of his ninetieth birthday. Guy's overall health has been good, and for much of the last twelve years he has been the primary caregiver for Kandy's mother (who is also named Mary, by the way). Guy and Mary have been married forty years. Mary suffers from dementia and her disease is advancing rapidly. She is dependent on Guy for help with the activities of daily living and intermittently dependent on support from their daughters, including Kandy. Mary and Guy each had children before they married and share one child, Nikki, who is the youngest of the combined five girls.

When Guy became acutely ill, he was hospitalized with a preliminary diagnosis of pancreatic disease – possibly pancreatic cancer. He was stabilized and a stent placed in his liver. During his hospital stay, Mary's world came tumbling down. She became very confused. Kandy and her sisters felt their world shake as well. Who could provide daily care for Mom? What would happen to their dad? He was to return home until biopsies could be performed.

No one in their family could have imagined Guy and Mary not in their beautiful, old home. No one could have imagined them living separately. But, for now, this housing arrangement is working.

Guy presented Kandy and her family with what appeared to be a stubborn and self-centered decision. Instead of going to his and Mary's home of forty-plus years, he insisted that he go to his oldest daughter Sherry's home. Kandy was shocked. She called me. How could he do this! We talked for a long time. I asked her if she thought Guy was scared. Could he be frightened about his health? Could he be afraid of what would happen to Mary if he did not survive? She wept as she realized that he was in pain and afraid. We talked about who would be his confidant. Who could this stalwart retired person turn to in his time of need?

When Guy was discharged, he moved to Sherry's house, and the family moved Mary from her home to live with Kay, Kandy's older sister. Guy was able to recuperate. Mary forgot quickly about the changes in her environment and loved when there were joint meals with Guy. She felt they were dating again. No one told her differently. Without the burden of Mary's care and knowing she was doing well with her daughter Kay, Guy was given an opportunity to make decisions about his own diagnosis, and ultimately, his own fate.

Several months have gone by. No one in their family could have imagined Guy and Mary not in their beautiful, old home. No one could have imagined them living separately. But, for now, this housing arrangement is working. Both Guy and Mary are getting exactly what they need in separate, loving environments. Home for Guy is with his oldest daughter; home for Mary is with Kay.

You will, of course, need to review and consider the long-term financial aspects of the housing arrangements your Mom and Dad require. This review cannot be avoided though in truth no one wants to touch this aspect of care for the aging, especially if family members do not fully understand their parents' financial picture. David's mother's care cost nearly a million dollars in the five years she had round-the-clock home care. This figure includes all her expenses, even her home insurance, utilities, medicines, home-health staff, and fees for the bank that oversaw the plan. Not until one of her trusts was completely depleted and the bank sent a notice that the family was $35,000 in arrears did the family, as a whole, fully understand how much their decision to keep Isabel at home had really cost.

Know the real cost of your options

Even if money is plentiful, we still have a duty and obligation to explore all options. David and I often wondered if he and his family might be neglecting some of their responsibilities by insisting that Isabel live in her own home, regardless of the costs. Were they only responsible for the health aspects of their mother's care or were they avoiding other duties by keeping her at home? More money could have been accessed in Isabel's case, but David took the bank's note as a "wake-up" call – as time to consider and present to his siblings alternatives to independent living for their mother. Assisted living seemed better able to provide the care and comfort that Isabel needed in her final struggle with Alzheimer's – and it was more cost-effective.

David's parents esteemed higher education and considered it an essential requirement for their children and grandchildren. Thus, after each of our three children was born, Ralph Emmott not only called to wish us well, but to make sure we had applied for the child's social security number. Before the children were even a month old, Ralph and Isabel had set up college accounts for them. But Ralph died in his early sixties, so several of those college funds for grandchildren were not completed and others were never started. During the spending of Isabel's estate, David often wondered if his Dad would have made different decisions. David felt strongly that Ralph and Isabel would have wanted to participate in all their grandchildren's higher education. In hindsight, David regrets that so much of the family's funds were spent so quickly and so unnecessarily to keep Isabel at home. It's not that he selfishly wanted any of the funds; he merely wanted to care for his mother appropriately while being respectful of his family's hard-earned, life savings.

My mother's situation was pretty straightforward. She had little to no money. The small amount of money she had after divorcing my dad ran out very quickly. For many years, Mom worked to supplement her social security income, but as she aged and could no longer work, her choices for where she would live narrowed. Mom would need to live with one of her ten children or reside in a place that honored Medicare insurance or Medicaid benefits or both.

In the chapter on goals of care (chapter 6), I described how my family recognized that Mother's care needs exceeded Cinda and her family's ability to care for her in their home. Cinda and I carefully sought out other living situations that would meet our mother's healthcare needs. Mom was still of sound mind but we felt we should research her options before presenting them to her. We quickly discovered that assisted living was not covered by the resources we had at our disposal.

As we visited long-term care facilities (skilled nursing homes), we were devastated that so few were available. Our experience underscores how important it is to determine what actual arrangements are available to your family and in your community. Regardless of the list you glean from community resources or the large promises

Many of these places could take good care of Mom's physical health and fit our financial constraints, but they failed to be what Mom would need socially and psychologically.

that will be made to you by facility marketers, the only way to make an informed decision is to investigate each facility for yourself. You need to know the location of each place and what it looks, feels, and smells like. The location of the facility is immensely important because you or some other trusted family member should be able to visit the facility easily and often.

Cinda and I visited at least a dozen places in the Kansas City area during step three in our process. In step one, we considered Mom's health status. Her primary health problems were failing sight and hearing, hypertension, and chronic back pain, which made walking painful and unstable. Our concerns centered mostly on nutrition, hygiene, and safety. We knew all too well what her financial situation looked like (step two). Mom's place of residence would have to be a facility that accepted Medicare and Medicaid. We quickly learned that only progressive or skilled nursing facilities fell into that category.

We did not find one place that fit Mom's situation, even though I personally knew staff who worked at some of them. Many of these places could take good care of Mom's physical health and fit our financial constraints, but they failed to be what Mom would need socially and psychologically. She was quite social, at that time, and an avid reader of books and newspapers. Asking our mother to live where the majority of the residents were mentally and physically compromised didn't seem like a good choice.

Each time we visited a new place we would venture into its assisted-living area. It was different from the skilled nursing area; it had less moaning, fewer unpleasant odors, and fewer wheelchairs lined up in the hall with debilitated residents nodding off. There were libraries, people playing Bingo, and beauty parlors that were actually being used. And, most of all, assisted living areas provide ways for residents to exercise their autonomy through larger rooms, flexible eating times, ability to come and go with friends and relatives, and even drive. Assisted living seemed the best option for us, but, we had no funding to accommodate increasing levels of assistance.

> *When Mom walked into the entry of the old church, her face lit up. She loved the Western décor. ... She couldn't wait to make new friends and have her own space again.*

One day when visiting a state-subsidized long-term care facility about twenty miles from Kansas City, a social worker mentioned a very small, assisted-living facility a short distance away. She said it was owned by a couple she knew and that they were state approved for some funding. Cinda and I immediately went to see this facility.

We pulled up in the parking lot of what had probably been a church at one time. The building itself was not extremely inviting or sophisticated in appearance. We walked into an interior room interestingly decorated in a Western style. There we saw men and women, similar in appearance to our mother, chatting, watching television, and interacting in a large, open room. Large windows covered the entire back of the room where a dining hall appeared. No urine stench. No wheelchair line. Music played. There was energy. We could feel it.

After talking with the two owners, we found out that the state maintained a waiting list for assisted care that already had 800 names on it. We found out as well that care for Mom in this facility would be $2,000 per month, if paid for privately. In talking with the facility's social worker, we learned that people on the waiting list could move to the top of the list if they began as private pay. If they then became unable to sustain the charges, they could apply for financial assistance (Medicaid). We were more than intrigued.

On our drive home, we considered how many of Mable's children, our siblings, might pitch in monthly, even if only for a few months. Cinda made a few phone calls. I talked to David to see what amount we might absorb of the $2,000 each month. We were so surprised at the generosity of our siblings. Seven of the ten of us offered to contribute for a period of ninety days to test drive the situation if Mom agreed.

When Mom visited the assisted-living residence, I think that bells in heaven were ringing. Recall that my mother spent much of her time in rural Oklahoma and in church settings, no less. When Mable walked into the entry of the old church, her face lit up. She loved the Western decor. She thought the individual rooms were huge. She couldn't wait to make new friends and have her own space again. We talked about furniture. She asked if she could have her own little refrigerator. It was magical.

Ninety days went by. Generous support flowed from Mable's children. One of our sisters even saved her tips and sent them to Cinda whenever she could. We were able to buy Mom new clothes and even had cable television added to her room. Finally, after six months, she was approved for state assistance. O, happy day! We had already experienced moving Mom from her rental house to Cinda's and from Cinda's to assisted living. And we did it without compromising Mom's health needs or getting into financial difficulties. Because Mom's life had been demanding, she was easily pleased at this stage, and all of us felt good about the choice.

Justice vs. autonomy

During my formal training to assist families and healthcare professionals make decisions in hospital settings, I was taught that there were four primary principles that should guide the decision-making process: autonomy, beneficence, nonmaleficence, and justice. Bioethicists Tom Beauchamp and Jim Childress had proposed these principles as a practical way to deal with complex healthcare decisions.

For much of my career as a nurse ethicist, I viewed autonomy as the trump card for all healthcare decisions. Essentially, I believed that personal decisions were just that: personal. If good medical choices were presented to capable individuals, they would weigh the risks and benefits and self-direct their care. And if anyone had an explicit loss of capacity, a next-of-kin or an appointed healthcare proxy could make substituted decisions for their loved ones.

How simple, I frequently thought. But questions about where Mom or Dad should live have wide impact and affect many people whose opinions must also be considered. Therefore, in all cases involving decisions about where your loved ones should live, the principle of autonomy should be balanced with justice. Justice involves choosing what is fair and equitable to the person being cared for and the people caring for them.

In the opening paragraphs of this chapter, I introduced you to my friend Judy and her husband Charlie and their efforts to help Judy's mom find a new place to live. Remember that Marjorie's health is stable and she takes only one medication, despite having celebrated her ninety-fifth birthday. She has memory issues, but does not appear to have dementia. She uses a walker to go long distances but is generally sure-footed. She has Medicare and her personal finances are abundant. Her situation is one that many of us would yearn for at step three: In what community and in what kind of facility should Marjorie choose to live?

> *Justice involves choosing what is fair and equitable to the person being cared for and the people caring for them.*

When Judy asked her mother about moving to Kansas City, Marjorie replied, "I wouldn't be opposed to it. I would like to be closer to you." Judy was thrilled and literally jumped on her mother's response. She was fearful that if she hesitated, Marjorie would change her mind.

Visits to several independent living, assisted living, and long-term care facilities gave both Judy and Charlie many acceptable choices within a few miles' drive from their home in Mission Hills, Kansas. One day when Judy and I were together, I overheard her say that she and Charlie were meeting someone who was going to show them a new assisted living development near where they lived. I offered to go with them. The facility was as I expected it would be: not quite finished, very lovely, and shown to us by an energetic marketing representative.

I encouraged Judy to look past the beauty and the newness of the place and to ask the marketing representative questions regarding additional expenses for helping with the activities of daily living. There are usually daily charges for each additional activity for which help is provided, such as reminding one to take medicines, helping one get dressed, or assisting residents to the dining room. Other charges can also escalate, such as changing soiled linens more than once a week. I encouraged Judy to envision the place with fifty residents, Marjorie possibly being at the high end of functionality. And, lastly, I asked the representative if her corporation worked with hospice organizations when serious illness occurs. She didn't know, but promised to check with other homes that the corporation owned.

> *The last thing I suggested to Judy as she got out of the car was that she ask herself which of their options would ensure that she could someday look back without regrets.*

When we left the construction site, I drove Judy and Charlie home. Charlie entered their house, and Judy stayed behind. I asked Judy what she was thinking. She thought for a moment and shared how her mother was so cooperative and willing to move from Salina to Kansas City. She further shared how big her mother's independent townhouse was in Salina and how well she was doing in many ways, except for loneliness. Judy said she really believed her mom deserved to live independently. She sighed.

The last thing I suggested to Judy as she got out of the car was that she ask herself which of their options would ensure that she could someday look back without regrets. She paused thoughtfully, then shot me a grin and said, "I think I've made my mind up."

That conversation occurred several months ago. Marjorie moved to Kansas City to a one bedroom, independent living residence that is part of an entire continuum of long-term care. Judy and Charlie have an on-site back-up plan for assisted living and even skilled care. No more urgent calls from Marjorie. But if she does call, Judy and Charlie are only two miles from Marjorie's new home. Marjorie is enjoying her independence and frequent outings with her family. Judy is planning on having a much delayed orthopedic surgery on an old knee injury. Charlie and Judy are planning a river cruise in Amsterdam this fall. There is temporary peace for all the family: justice has occurred for all.

Lessons for Living without Regrets

- Deciding where your parents will live in their declining years is emotionally and ethically challenging with no right answers.

- It is essential to include your parents in this discussion and help them overcome any fears that may be inhibiting their participation.

- To make the best decision for your family, consider your parents health status, your family's financial resources, and the housing options available in your community.

- A final question to ask yourself regarding your decision is: "Which decision is best for my parents and fair to everyone?"

CHAPTER 9

Healthcare Treatment Directives
Guidance for Proxy Decision Makers

In an earlier chapter, I referred to advance care planning as a huge umbrella that covers many things regarding one's life values, financial estate, and two basic questions in the healthcare arena: "Who will make my healthcare decisions when I cannot?" "What healthcare treatments do I want to receive or not receive when I am seriously ill?" In Choosing a Healthcare Proxy (chapter 4), I focused on the "who" question and urged you and your parents to record your choice of proxies on the document called the Durable Power of Attorney for Healthcare. If you were not convinced by that chapter of how important that document is, I hope that you will be by the end of this chapter.

Our focus in this chapter is on how you and your parents can make known your specific wishes regarding future healthcare treatments. This second part of advance care planning is called a Medical Treatment or Healthcare Treatment Directive. You may have heard it referred to as a "living will." It is called "living" because individuals are living when they make their choices known (when the will is read, so to speak). And it is called "will" because your parents are testifying about the medical

> *Healthcare Treatment Directives are intended to serve as a guide or roadmap to those who will make decisions for others.*

treatments they want to have done or not done to them when they can no longer communicate these decisions and desires. Healthcare Treatment Directives are intended to serve as a guide or roadmap to those who will make decisions for others. This directive, like the durable power of attorney or proxy choice, becomes effective whenever a person loses his or her capacity to make decisions.

A brief personal history

If I had written this book as early as five years ago, I would have written this chapter addressing medical directives first. I would have begun with the history of advance care planning and simply assumed that you and your parents were eager to hear about your right to direct your own healthcare and that you were literally dying (no pun intended) to consider your options and document them for future use. What, then, changed my mind?

Recently over a glass of wine, and after we had completed several sessions with a financial advisor, David and I set aside our financial goals to share personal feelings, review our past frustrations and successes, and plan our future. I told David that I now felt that much of my two decades of work in healthcare ethics had been futile: "All that damn work on advance directives," I said sadly. By this I meant my efforts to champion the entire umbrella of advance care planning, especially the healthcare directive component.

I thought back over my long experience with the bioethics center in Kansas City (now called the Center for Practical Bioethics). We not only pioneered advance care planning, we also wrote and refined a workbook about advance care planning called *Caring Conversations*® and held workshops in Kansas City showing families how to use the workbook. We also trained trainers across the nation to hold their own advance care planning seminars. We thought that everyone would be eager to appoint a proxy and share his or her list of "do's" and "don'ts" regarding end-of-life treatments. Feeding tube or not? Breathing machine, yes or no? Dialysis? Hospitalization or hospice care? Documenting these decisions was easy, logical, and empowering or so we thought, and we were absolute zealots!

Choosing the right person (healthcare proxy) is important, but we truly believed that documenting one's wishes was the absolute best way to prevent bad things from happening when a patient is unable to communicate. Staff at the ethics center knew many families in our community who had not chosen an individual to speak for their moms or dads and whose parents had not documented their preferences about how they wanted to be treated during times of illness and frailty. Their healthcare decisions had become painful tugs-of-war between family members (primarily adult children) and physicians. Family members and individual patients had to endure aggressive, often futile, treatment, sometimes resulting in a state of medical limbo. Despite our best efforts and enthusiasm, families were not prepared. Were they unaware of their rights? Did they not care about this issue? Or was something else inhibiting them?

> *Choosing the right person (healthcare proxy) is important, but we truly believed that documenting one's wishes was the absolute best way to prevent bad things from happening when a patient is unable to communicate.*

Year after year, we tried various approaches and tweaked the documents: we worked in our local community, joined or founded national coalitions, sat on national boards, and worked with citizens and professionals. The very premise of the *Caring Conversations* program was to promote self-reflection for individuals so that they could appoint a proxy, share their wishes with that person and subsequently with their healthcare providers. The booklets began

Colby contends that when families are reluctant or hesitant to make decisions, well-intended doctors will do their best work to keep the patient alive without regard for the kind of treatment the patient might actually want.

with guided conversations about one's past experience and values, and then introduced the notion of healthcare treatments and decisions and, as a last step, asked individuals to complete the two documents verifying their choice of proxy and specifying the

medical treatments they desired during serious illness or their final period of dying. The documents, we believed, would tie up all those loose ends that often create chaos when family members are clueless about their loved one's wishes. When serious illness deprives a person of his or her ability to make cognitive decisions, the proxy or other family members must already know what the person's living will or advance directive contains. It is, and it seemed, that simple to us.

Throughout these years, we learned a truth that my friend and colleague, Bill Colby, wrote about in his 2006 book, *Unplugged*. Colby, the lawyer who took the Nancy Cruzan case to the U.S. Supreme Court, claims that, most of the time, families don't really want to talk, think, or make healthcare choices when family members are hospitalized. He confirms what research reveals about dying in America. Most of us die in one of three ways: from cancer, heart and lung disease, or old age. The latter is often preceded by frailty, loss of independence, and dementia, but on all three paths medical teams and families have choices to make, though family members and healthcare providers are reluctant to make these decisions.

The world that *Caring Conversations* assumed was the polar opposite of Colby's depiction of what really happens during hospitalizations. He contends that when families are reluctant or hesitant to make decisions, well-intended doctors will do their best work to keep the patient alive without regard for the kind of treatment the patient might actually want. In the end, a type of hospital culture or medical glide path takes over and a typical standard of care or aggressive medical model of care begins. In cases involving aging patients, a less aggressive model of care may be more fitting. The focus should be family centered and shift toward comfort care, that is, toward alleviating pain and other symptoms. Such an approach, often referred to as palliative care in hospitals or hospice care in other settings, may be more in keeping with the patient's wishes than an effort to use all available technology to prolong life.

If individuals in the very midst of healthcare decisions hesitate to participate in such deliberations, it is no wonder that efforts to encourage advance planning so often fell on deaf ears. We also learned that professionals, especially physicians, are not trained to share decisions. They are trained to save lives. At best, about a third of all adults complete advance care documents, and even then, these documents are rarely consulted when patients most need them. Our community didn't fully embrace advance care planning and neither did our nation.

> *In cases involving aging patients, a less aggressive model of care may be more fitting. The focus should be family centered and shift toward comfort care, that is, toward alleviating pain and other symptoms.*

Conversations and documents about medical decisions did not solve the problems I experienced as an Intensive Care nurse or change the stories that ethics center staff were told by anguished and frustrated families in our community.

"I'm worn out with it," I said to David, while sipping my wine. "It doesn't work."

Avoiding the medical glide path

So why am I writing this chapter? What can I tell you to help you and your parents prepare for illness and dying so that your parents' dying will be expressive of their lives and not simply another cookie-cutter death like the ones Colby describes as occurring on the typical medical glide path?

In his books, Colby refers extensively to two very high-profile cases that are exceptions to what usually happens. Nancy Cruzan was injured in a car wreck in 1983. Her family waited for her capacity (and consciousness) to return, but when it was clear that her condition was irreversible they sought to have medical treatment withdrawn. The family was sure that Nancy would not have chosen treatment that had no benefit to her. The Missouri court refused to allow the treatment to be withdrawn because the state of Missouri had no clear and convincing evidence that this is what Nancy herself would have chosen. When Colby argued the case before the U.S. Supreme Court, the justices agreed with the state's right to clear and convincing evidence of Nancy's wishes but also upheld the individual's right to refuse any medical treatment. Once the state was presented with clear and convincing evidence of Nancy's choice, her family was able to get the treatment discontinued and Nancy died eleven days later on December 26, 1990.

Theresa Marie or "Terri" Schiavo suffered massive brain damage following a complete cardiac arrest in her home in 1990.

After several months in a coma, she was diagnosed as being in a permanent vegetative state. Attempts to bring her to awareness were futile. In 1998, her husband sought to have her life support removed on grounds that Terri would not have chosen to continue treatment with no hope of recovery. He was opposed by her parents who continued to hope that she would get better. A series of court hearings ensued, and Terri's treatment was further compromised by the controversy. Finally, all appeals were exhausted, and Terri's husband was able to direct that her treatment be discontinued. She died on March 31, 2005.

Nancy Cruzan and Terri Schiavo were both young when they were incapacitated, and their incapacity persisted for years. Both women had families who cared greatly for them and wanted a say in their treatment. Both families also had strong opinions about the kind of treatments their loved one would have chosen. These extreme cases help us understand why it is so important for families to know their loved ones' wishes and to participate in helping them choose the healthcare treatments most

Advance Directives serve to empower families engaged in caregiving; they can also give healthcare providers the comfort of knowing that they are talking to the right people.

likely to achieve their goals. Nancy's and Teri's youth reminds us that although this book is meant to assist families with aging parents, all of us need advance directives. Advance Directives serve to empower families engaged in caregiving; they can also give healthcare providers the comfort of knowing that they are talking to the right people.

The older one is, the more likely it is that family and proxies will need to make and communicate that person's healthcare decisions. But no matter how old a person is, being able to make the best choices for a loved one is profoundly important and diffi-cult. Families may be reluctant to get involved initially, especially in acute care settings, but over time, as acute situations become chronic conditions, there is no escaping the responsibility to advo-cate for a vulnerable or totally dependent family member. And, as the Cruzan and Schiavo cases demonstrate, families must some-times advocate for discontinuing treatments that over time have proven futile.

The Cruzan family was so convinced that their daughter should have the right to die that they spent years before the Missouri and federal courts, including the U.S. Supreme Court. Terri Schiavo's parents, unlike Nancy Cruzan's, continued to hope that their daugh-ter's health would improve even though she was in a coma for more than ten years. They vehe-mently opposed her husband's view that Terri herself would not want to continue to receive nutritional support since this treatment was only prolonging her death. As neither family had any written documentation of their daughter's choices, the

The question at the heart of both cases was what the two young women would have said about the quality of their lives and future if they had been able to speak for themselves.

question at the heart of both cases was what the two young women would have said about the quality of their lives and future if they had been able to speak for themselves. How would these young women have defined the quality of their lives and what would they have chosen for their future? These are the same questions that you must ask yourself when you are considering healthcare options with and for your parents.

Facing the unimaginable

A short time ago I was asked to speak to an assembly of healthcare professionals about what I had learned about decision making from my patients. I talked about my nursing education and subsequent experience as an ICU nurse. I confessed that after less than ten years in pediatric and adult ICUs I frequently asked myself "Am I in the wrong profession?" "Do I work for the wrong organization?" "Am I a bad nurse?"

Much later I learned that the reason I was so perplexed was that, by training and environment, I was working in a caring profession that focused primarily on the physical aspects of curing. We really didn't want to know much about our patients' wishes and worked much more fluidly when their families remained in the waiting room. We were trained to manage multiple tubes, machines, monitors, inputs and outputs, and to record all this "caring" in patients' charts. We were not trained to manage our patients' healthcare choices or help them face the unimaginable. The ten minutes on the even hours when families came into our intensively focused rooms were dreaded, even by kind-hearted, well-trained, well-meaning nurses.

The most frustrating part of my career as a nurse and ethicist was watching families and patients face difficult decisions regarding their loved ones. They easily submitted to a medical approach when they or a family member became seriously ill. That is, they submitted to "dying on an institutional glide path," as Bill Colby puts it, letting well-intended healthcare providers focus on extending their loved ones' lives no matter how dire the situation. Of course, extending life is not always a bad thing. Life is good, even precious, and should be followed by a good death. What is bad is allowing an impersonal, mechanized, routine medical culture take over the lives of those who are depending on us to be their advocates. Should we allow our mothers and fathers to die institutional deaths in hospital environments, often isolated from us and other loved ones? I don't think so.

I recall taking care of an elderly man in the medical ICU for more than two weeks. He had suffered a severe stroke and was intubated upon arrival to the hospital and transferred to my unit. His prognosis was, I could only guess, very grim. I was not certain, because even though I was his primary nurse for seven, twelve-hour shifts, the possibility of his dying was never shared with me or discussed with his family. His wife visited every day. She dressed in a St. John knit suit, wore gloves, and, occasionally, a hat. She was lovely. She was worried. She herself was quite frail. The second week of my caring for him, she asked me if I could pull a chair into the room for her.

> *Extending life is not always a bad thing. Life is good, even precious, and should be followed by a good death. What is bad is allowing an impersonal, mechanized, routine medical culture take over the lives of those who are depending on us to be their advocates.*

I was stunned. My colleagues and I had been so intent on taking care of our patient's physical needs, we had not even noticed that his loving wife had no place to sit during her visits. Do you wonder that I began to question my career choice? I knew that this narrow focus on keeping the patient alive was something less than a wholehearted attempt to really care for patients and their families. We weren't giving patients and their families a chance to participate in decision making. We didn't even give them a chair in the room, let alone at the table where decisions were being made. We thought we knew what was best for them.

Our focus was clearly directed at the health of our patients, at extending and prolonging life. But weren't we neglecting something else: the values that promote human dignity? Only later, while studying healthcare ethics and working at a bioethics center did I realize that my long-standing professional and personal discomfort stemmed from not knowing that tending to the unique wishes of my patients is as important as newfound surgical techniques, medications, and the life-sustaining procedures that define hospital intensive care units. Ignoring patients' values and their families was a large part of my distress. Patients' wishes and beliefs should have been integrated, intertwined, with the treatments that my colleagues and I mistook for total care.

I wasn't the only nurse who was restless. Many of us experienced symptoms that several years later were referred to as "moral distress." We weren't bad nurses; we were good nurses who wanted to be better. But we didn't know how. Not only did we have to learn the importance of attending to our patients' wishes, so did our patients and their friends and families. Everyday citizens with no medical background needed to prepare to sit with white coats when decisions about life and death were being made. Their loved ones, especially their aging parents, were counting on them. They should have demanded this privilege long ago, but they were unprepared to participate fully in the decisions.

Advance Directives reimagined

As I confessed to David that I was done providing workbooks and seminars for families and equally worn out from educating nurses and physicians in end-of-life decision making, deep down I realized that there has to be a reason why advance care planning isn't being embraced by families and professionals, especially in cases involving aging persons. So what is it that I really want to say before

I hang up my coat forever? Do I have any sacred words that will convince you and future generations of the value of advance care planning? I think so.

Earlier in this book, I implored each of us to choose and document a healthcare proxy. I stand by that. Your healthcare proxy will not only advocate for desired treatments but he or she can also reject undesired treatments. Rarely will you find an aging and frail parent who "wants everything done" to prolong life regardless of its quality. Remember that part of my mother's newfound autonomy included preparing the family for her death by telling us that she was not worried about healthcare treatments as such, but by treatments that might be unnecessary – that might better be withheld. That was not something our family had expected her to say.

My mother's first attempt to do her advance care planning consisted of completing two documents. They were called "terminal condition" and "permanently unconscious" declarations. I still have these two documents, dated 1988. An attorney prepared the documents and witnessed them. For the "terminal condition" documents to become effective, a person had to have a condition that was considered terminal (defined as expecting death within six months). Only in that case, could a treatment be discontinued. The "permanently unconscious" document allowed for stopping treatments only if the person was unconscious and treatments would not alleviate pain. Unfortunately, these types of

The Patient Self-Determination Act gave all Americans the constitutional right to appoint a proxy and to describe in writing or orally what treatments they did or did not wish to have when they became unable to make decisions about their health and healthcare.

documents were useless when patients had illnesses or injuries that resulted in severe chronic conditions that fell outside the categories of cancer or coma, such as persons who suffer from major, debilitating strokes or from serious illness and frailty at the end of life. Some people argued, for example, that Nancy Cruzan and Terri Schiavo were not terminal, as they could have lived indefinitely with nutritional support.

Ten years later, Mom updated her living will or advance care plan. This was a few years after the Patient Self-Determination Act gave all Americans the constitutional right to appoint a proxy and to describe in writing or orally what treatments they did or did not wish to have when they became unable to make decisions about their health and healthcare. By appointing her son-in-law, my husband David, as her documented healthcare proxy, she made him her decision maker in the event that she lost capacity or the ability to make her own healthcare decisions, regardless of whether her underlying condition was terminal or not.

She also made it quite clear in conversation and by completing a healthcare treatment directive document that should she ever become seriously ill she did not want life-prolonging interventions. She directed instead that her doctor turn from aggressive curative treatments to comfort care. She wanted hospice care if receiving it would not create an undue burden on my sister with whom she was living at the time she documented her wishes. Thus, my mom's planning encompassed every contingency. She completed both advance care documents; that is, she appointed a proxy and specified her wishes regarding medical care if she were to become seriously ill and incapacitated. She didn't need to have cancer or be in a coma to have her wishes honored.

Using my mother's experience as a model, here are four things you can do to help your parents accomplish an end-of-life plan. First, get updated on what has or hasn't already been talked about, agreed to, and documented. Check to see if your parents are holding onto a terminal condition or permanently unconscious declaration. Those documents are outdated and pretty useless. They should be replaced.

Second, make sure that your parent or parents have chosen and documented a healthcare proxy. Review the life lessons in chapter four to help you and your parents process their choice. Remind them that elder spouses can become frail and unable to advocate for each other and that a spouse may even die before he or she can exercise the other's proxy. This reality is not easy to face, but use their friends as examples. It is quite likely that they have already witnessed a husband or wife being suddenly left with no one to advocate for him or her.

Aging parents may also believe that the eldest son should be the legal decision maker or that their appointed estate trustee or lawyer will make their healthcare decisions. Such choices often lead to chaos and conflict. Though my mother had ten living children, she chose my husband as her healthcare proxy. At first several of my sisters were shocked. Then we realized that she trusted David, a physician, to understand the nature of her healthcare decisions. She also knew that he would consult with all her

The proxy performs a specific role in protecting your loved ones' autonomy. However, he or she does not supplant the family and will need the entire family's support.

children but ultimately endure the challenges better than her own, sentimental children. Clarifying these things while your parents are well can help you and your siblings understand their choices, decrease chances of hurt feelings, and allow for a deeper understanding of important issues.

Third, eliminate the mystery and myths surrounding proxy or surrogate decision making by asking your parents today or as soon as possible to complete the Durable Power of Attorney for Healthcare Decisions. Make sure that they designate a proxy, and whenever possible, be sure to document an alternate. Be realistic about this: according to current data, 85 percent of us will experience some kind of incapacity or dementia that will make it impossible for us to advocate for ourselves.

Having an informed healthcare proxy present and ready to partner with the family and healthcare team is the best chance anyone has to insure that his or her wishes will be honored and that he or she will experience a decent and humane death.

Fourth, and finally, be prepared to support and help your parents' chosen proxies as they prepare to step into your parents' shoes and be their voice. The proxy performs a specific role in protecting your loved ones' autonomy. However, he or she does not supplant the family and will need the entire family's support. Having an informed healthcare proxy present and ready to partner with the family and healthcare team is the best chance anyone has to insure that his or her wishes will be honored and that he or she will experience a decent and humane death.

Using healthcare directives to discuss clinical scenarios and treatment options

The medical or healthcare treatment directive instructs or guides your proxy. It answers the second of our two questions, namely, "What healthcare treatments do I want to receive or not receive when I am seriously ill? This document gives individuals an opportunity to consent to certain treatments and refuse others when a healthcare problem results in their inability to make or convey decisions. But treatment directives, as ethicists in Kansas City and our nation imagined, are at the core of the very reason I have been so frustrated by this work. The reason for my distress is simple: no one, not even well-trained, experienced physicians, can predict the many clinical situations that a serious illness may produce. There are few, if any, clearly predictable "if-then" situations during serious illness. Thus, individuals may know their end-of-life wishes and still have a hard time conveying the essence of those decisions in a document.

But that doesn't mean that we shouldn't complete the healthcare directive. I have come to believe that a healthcare treatment directive will serve you and your parents best if and only if you approach this document as a tool, that is, as more of a conversational piece than as objective instructions. Here's how I think it should work: Have your parents choose a healthcare proxy, and discuss their wishes with him or her, using the healthcare treatment directive as a guide to discussion. Then when serious illness or incapacity occurs, the proxy and healthcare team can assess the clinical situation and discuss in depth the interventions that are commonly used to treat persons in this condition and determine which of these interventions is most appropriate to meet your parents' wishes and goals of care.

> *individuals may know their end-of-life wishes and still have a hard time conveying the essence of those decisions in a document.*

What I am suggesting is that the treatment directive be used primarily to help you and your parents discuss possible clinical scenarios. The guidance you are looking for concerns the treatments they would want their proxy to consider should they encounter similar circumstances. Three major areas of medical treatment are covered in most healthcare treatment directive documents: hydration (when one is too ill or compromised to swallow enough fluids to maintain healthy hydration, an intravenous line can be used); nutrition (when one is too ill to consume adequate nutrition by mouth, an intravenous line or feeding tube can be inserted); and oxygenation (when one cannot breath adequately to maintain blood oxygen levels, nasal oxygen can be delivered and/or tubes into trachea and lungs can be used with ventilators).

Other medical interventions addressed in a treatment document often include kidney dialysis and use of antibiotics. You, your parents, and the healthcare proxy also need to consider whether your parents would consent to or want these treatments tried on a temporary basis or put permanently in place. Discussions about these topics generally center on what your parents deem as an acceptable quality of life. Don't let the terms or topics frighten you, or you won't be prepared for the issues you will face. Consider the following example.

Mrs. Johnson wrote on her treatment directive that she would not want artificial nutrition if she has no hope of regaining her prior state of health. Now she has had a stroke and is unable to swallow. She rehabilitates well in many ways but swallowing continues to be difficult and she remains confused. The neurologist anticipates that she will improve in areas of eating and communicating and talks to a surgeon about placing a feeding tube (PEG tube) so that she can be transported to a rehabilitation facility.

Mrs. Johnson's healthcare treatment directive clearly states that she doesn't want a feeding tube. However, in this situation, no one knows what her condition will look like when all is said and done. Will she return to her prior healthcare status and quality of life? It is unclear. A healthcare proxy can partner with the healthcare team to determine how the unanticipated "gray" areas in Mrs. Johnson's clinical situation affect her decisions. Based on this discussion, they might agree to a feeding tube for a limited amount of time with plans to withdraw the tube if there is no improvement in her condition. Or they might reinforce the instructions written on the directive and reject the placing of a feeding tube. Decisions like this one are very challenging, but they are not unique to Mrs. Johnson's family. Each day, all across our nation, some individual or family faces similar choices.

These gray areas are the very reason that so many physicians and families argue against the use of treatment directives. But my experience tells me that when a chosen healthcare agent is present, especially if in-depth conversations about these topics have occurred, a good decision will result. If you think that you or your parent's proxy is not confident or knowledgeable enough to begin or sustain conversations about these topics, help is available. The *Caring Conversations* program that I worked on at the Center for Practical Bioethics has been updated and is extremely helpful in processing medical interventions. In fact, only two years ago, major changes were made in the program specifically to help the healthcare proxy discuss healthcare treatments. It is most important, however, to consider your parent's disease and diagnosis. What do individual treatment options accomplish and do they fit your parent's current situation, goals and values? That is, do they contribute to your parent's goals of care and quality of life?

Recall that in chapter six, we discussed questions that can help you help your parents establish goals of care. These same questions can help guide your decisions in critical moments. I suggested in another chapter that you need to search for the things you *should* do, not for everything you *could* do. Your parent's critical moments should be treated in the same spirit as he or she has lived. Recall, too, that each decision has a domino effect: if you decide for or against a particular treatment, what decision will you face next? For instance, if you begin a treatment, such as a feeding tube, on a temporary or trial basis, and Mom or Dad doesn't improve, can you withdraw that treatment easily? Different states have different regulations on withdrawing a medical treatment; if your state doesn't allow for the tube's withdrawal, are you willing to agree to a permanent tube for nutritional support?

Medical teams and state institutions will usually err on the side of life. You or your parents' proxies must integrate your parents' values and wishes into decisions of care. Be prepared, as advocates, to grind your heels in, if necessary.

My husband David and his older brother Cameron were co-guardians of their mother's estate and co-proxies for her health-care decisions. Their decisions were not always exactly what some of Isabel's healthcare providers in her small town expected, especially her psychiatrist. Isabel experienced a decade of failing health that began with early-onset dementia, and her health and living arrangements changed many times and required many, sometimes agonizing, decisions. However, in the end, Isabel could not swallow. Nutrition and hydration were a final concern. Based on documentation and conversations it was clear that Isabel had strictly rejected the insertion of a feeding tube. That is, she had made it known that she did not want to undergo this medical treatment. I do not believe that David or his brother ever considered it, but if some of Isabel's providers had expected it as part of her treatment, having the document would have been essential. In applying what they see as the standard of care, medical teams and state institutions will usually err on the side of life. You or your parents' proxies must integrate your parents' values and wishes into decisions of care. Be prepared, as advocates, to grind your heels in, if necessary.

I have been involved in healthcare in some capacity for a very long time, since before I graduated from high school, and I have seen many changes. For many, many years I saw doctors treated as though they were gods and patients submitting to whatever they were told. I have seen families suffer in the waiting rooms of ICUs while their babies and aging parents were treated to invasive treatments without their voices being heard or attention being paid to what their lives would be like after treatment. My colleagues and I certainly hoped for something different than those scenarios.

Consider yourself part of the team so that you can give and take information. Learn what the clinicians' intentions are and teach them who your loved one is.

We worked hard as nurses, many times without the knowledge needed to get our patients and their families better positioned to share decisions. Sometimes we did get families involved and patient's heard; other times, we failed. We also saw that allowing the pendulum to swing too far in our effort to avoid paternalistic practices could also put patients and their families into situations that they were ill-prepared to handle, in many ways forcing them to bear the full responsibility of medical decision making.

My experience taught me three things that can prevent families and patients from coming up on the wrong side of a bad coin toss. First, be prepared. Know who the spokesperson – the proxy – is for the one who is seriously ill, aging, and possibly dying. Encourage family members to help the proxy decision maker and trust his or her decisions. Second, engage in frequent conversations with your parents and families about their health and healthcare wishes. Have casual conversations but also serious discussions about possible clinical situations and share what you learn about your parents' views with others as frequently as you can. Third, work with each person on the healthcare team. Consider yourself part of the team so that you can give and take information. Learn what the clinicians' intentions are and teach them who your loved one is. Healthcare for an aging person is only as good as it is appropriate. What will the offered treatments accomplish at this time in your loved one's life? What can you teach physicians and nurses about your mom? About your dad?

The night I told David that I was finished with my work in healthcare end-of-life decision making, he grinned as he listened. He knew that I was blowing off a little steam but my caring about what does or doesn't happen to each person when he or she is dying, especially if that one is frail and aging, will not die before I do. And so this chapter, based on what does and doesn't work, sits near the end of this book on life lessons about dying well. When your turn comes, your goal will be to make decisions each day, one day at a time, based on what you know that day. What is the best choice for your mom or dad or other loved one?

When your turn comes, your goal will be to make decisions each day, one day at a time, based on what you know that day. What is the best choice for your mom or dad or other loved one?

What would he or she say to the healthcare team right now, in this situation? The answers to these questions should be both logical and loving, using good information but never straying too far from the wisdom of your heart.

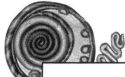

Lessons for Living without Regrets

● Using a healthcare treatment directive as a guide to discussions between your parents and their proxy is important. Such discussions help the proxy determine which medical interventions are appropriate, that is, which treatments fit your parents' wishes and goals.

● Be prepared to give and receive information with the healthcare team. Teach them who your loved one is.

● If your parents' values and healthcare preferences are unknown, a routine medical glide path will be used to determine your parents' medical treatment – one that will almost certainly include an aggressive approach to their end-of-life care.

● Family members and healthcare providers are often reluctant to make end-of-life decisions.

● Healthcare for aging persons is only as good as it is appropriate.

AFTERWORD

Son, Guardian, and Caregiver
A Doctor's Story

Death is inescapable, undeniable, and irrevocable. Inevitably, each of us will depart this world. And death is rarely pretty. How the drama plays itself out, however, can often be influenced and to some extent managed by those of us who care for dying loved ones. This book is a patchwork of how my wife and I tried to help our mothers and other dear friends depart this life with dignity and freedom from pain and fear. We didn't – and don't have – the perfect formula; we do not believe there is one. We certainly made mistakes along the way. But in these pages Helen has given readers a map marking some of the pitfalls we found along the trail. We hope that your trail will be purposeful, driven by compassion, and pure in its intent to honor your loved ones as they spend their final days, weeks, or years with you.

As I sat at my mother's funeral, I was overcome with intense loneliness, regret, and misgiving. Did she know that I wished I could have spent more time with her? Would she have approved of me taking vacation time and not coming to see her? My management of my mother's care was rough, especially when I attempted to include other family members in all my decisions. If I have a major regret, it is that the emotional impact of my mother's decline on my siblings and me added a fracture line to an already scattered family.

We did not hold hands and sing hymns at her bedside. There was no fairy-tale ending. We shared our loneliness separately, hoping that someday, the emptiness might drive us back together. In the meantime, we each wrestled with the reality of her decline and our conduct through her dying years. Death made us feel inept. Were we not prepared? Didn't we see it coming? Death exposed our denial and inability to grasp the obvious.

In many ways, death is the ultimate reality test. It rewards nobody and often makes fools of the rest of us. Who among us has not felt helpless when a loved one passes away while there we stand, holding a box of Kleenex in our hands? How many times have you heard, "I knew he was sick, but I didn't see it coming"? Some of us will hear the hoof-beats and be ready. Most of us won't. My hope and the hope embodied in this book is that all who have felt death's hammer will eventually recover from the blow, find a way to relieve the sense of guilt, and heal themselves and their families.

As a physician, I have seen end-of-life events unfolding from several unique perspectives. I have witnessed family members gripped in pain and sadness struggle to run interference and make weighty decisions about their parents' healthcare while also attempting to keep their individual lives from unraveling. Life is rugged and its last stages are usually the most complicated. I have now lived through my mother's death which was preceded by the decline of her mental faculties. I was initially alarmed and later heart-broken by my mother's loss of speech followed later by her inability to acknowledge or even recognize me. We would sometimes sit for hours in her den, sharing time together but no meaningful conversation. I struggled to accept the fact that she was not ever going to have a better day than yesterday and that the inevitability of her shrinking world was my new reality. That realization finally freed me to make a series of decisions that led to a smoother, more dignified transition for her.

I remember my wife telling me one evening, "Your mother chose you to be her guardian and durable power of attorney because she trusted you. You are not required to have consensus among your siblings. You are required to make appropriate and compassionate plans for her." Helen's words encouraged me to act more courageously.

Shortly after this pep talk, I moved my mother into an assisted-living facility. In the dead of winter, I wrapped her in her beautiful fur coat and carried her out to the car. I buckled her in and took her to her new home. My wife and kids had decorated her suite with as many of her favorite things as we could comfortably cram into it. Somberly, we left at dusk and drove home. There was nothing easy about moving her, but it was the right decision.

Isabel, my mother, was a grande dame. I always loved bringing my friends home to meet her because I knew they would inevitably exclaim, "Is that your mom? She's beautiful!" And she was. She always made me feel special, as she did all seven of her children. As we grew older, she made a point of staying involved in our lives.

Mom participated in my school activities, my athletics, and my personal life. I would have done anything to make her happy. She deserved it after raising us kids and facing the tragic aftermath of the brain injury that nearly blighted my oldest sister, Karen. To this day, Karen's incapacity is the singular devastating event that nearly destroyed my family. Yet, Isabel, the devoted and loving mother, mustered the grit to hold her head high and walk toward the future with fortitude and self-confidence, her entire family in tow. Her courageous leadership of our family remains unparalleled.

Do I have regrets? Sure, I do! I regret that I did not have more time with Mom when she was that bright light, when she was loving and affectionate, when she had her wit and wisdom. What I don't regret is that I was steadfast in communicating with her and her caregivers. Staying connected with those who spent part of every day with her was often all I could do, but with their help, I did my best to ensure her safety and to make her comfortable. I derived a sense of satisfaction knowing that she sensed she was receiving the best care available until her last breath.

Have you ever experienced something so tender and sweet that it leaves you dissolved in tears? The final scene of "Shenandoah," in which Jimmy Stewart, the patriarch of a Virginia family, is reunited with a son he thought had died in the Civil War, has that kind of warmth. The nakedness of the father's joy is penetratingly poignant. A similar richness attaches to the experience of caring for someone you love in their final days. Feeding my mother drops of water with a dropper and holding her delicate and beautiful hands in mine created that kind of joy. On those occasions, I wept like a baby. Such closeness is real and rare. It closes gaps between people while searing us with the realization that we will all share the same fate.

My advice to all who are given the responsibility to serve in this capacity is to seize the opportunity. It will bless their own lives to know that as they serve, they are being enriched. They are preserving a legacy while preparing their own.

Steve Jeffers, a dear friend and chaplain now deceased, once explained to me that grief is part of life and that we will continuously grieve losses, large and small, as we travel this world. When we are young, it may be the loss of a favorite shirt or a baseball glove. Later, it may be saying goodbye to a family pet or missing a free throw in a crucial game. And, finally, it may be saying goodbye to our friends and those we have loved longest: our parents. Identifying the emotional loss, understanding that it results from circumstances beyond our control, and making peace with it is part of healthy maturation. When one finally realizes that losses are an integral part of life, one can begin to accept that the world is full of unexpected downturns.

In our family, we called these downturns "life-lessons." One of my mother's favorite sayings when she caught one of us kids wallowing in self-pity, was, "Life is for the living! Get on with it!" Later, I saw the play, "Auntie Mame," and fell in love with her classic line, "All the world is a banquet, and half the sons-to-bitches are starving to death!"

My mom would have been a great Auntie Mame! She loved to entertain, dance, and converse. The truth, though, is that even if the world is a banquet, you will sometimes be served something that doesn't taste good or that is long past its expiration date. At such times, life reverts to being a cruel teacher, posing reality tests for the road ahead. To get on with life, we may need to see both sides.

If you are entering the role of caregiver, especially for a loved one, the humor and sadness intermingled in the stories in this book can help you know what to expect. There may be "aha" moments for you as you find commonalities between our experiences and your own. You will know, reading this book, that life gives as it takes away and that tears of joy and tears of sadness have the same flavor.

My dad's advice when one of us got knocked down was, "Pull yourself up! That's why they make bootstraps!" Being a decision maker and caregiver for many years for my mother, Helen's mother and, more recently, my sister Karen has required many a boot-strap tug. Make no mistake: caregiving is work – a labor of love for romantics, a debt of honor for others. But it can also be a remark-ably rewarding work.

Helen's and my ability to put our professional talents together to help our mothers in their declining days put us to the test. We managed to do it not because we were healthcare workers, but because we recognized that we had been a son and a daughter before we became a doctor and a nurse. And we were adult children before we became caregivers and in my case a guardian. We "descended" into our former roles as adult children in order to remain compassionate and caring. I learned that my job was to be an advocating son primarily and secondarily a physician. Keeping to this clear and simple formula helped me fulfill my role with more emotional honesty and satisfaction.

Every life is a unique journey. Human beings have tried for centuries to explain the meaning of life. As a physician I have learned that life is lived one day at a time without any guarantees or sureties. There is no such thing as security; there are only relative degrees of risk. Understanding and accepting that lives contract as frailties increase is the beginning of knowing how to help our parents and ourselves manage the aging process. Extreme age is often accompanied with increased medical needs and disabilities. Managing it well doesn't mean that we can avoid all the traps of aging, but it does mean that we can compensate to live with our changing circumstances.

So remain aware. Recognize that life is a continuum, and hasten to the side of those you love who are in need of what you alone can give them. Being close to loved ones while they are declining will open your heart and fill it even as it breaks.

David F. Emmott, MD
December 11, 2013